Case Studies for Pathophysiology

Case Studies for Pathophysiology

First Edition

Wei Li

University of Alabama at Birmingham

cognella
SAN DIEGO

Bassim Hamadeh, CEO and Publisher
Eric Kuntzman, Acquisitions Editor
Gem Rabanera, Senior Project Editor
Jeanine Rees, Production Editor
Juniper Perkins, Editorial Associate
JoHannah McDonald, Licensing Coordinator
Tiffany Mok, Senior Content Marketing Specialist
Natalie Piccotti, Director of Marketing
Kassie Graves, Senior Vice President, Editorial
Alia Bales, Director of Project Editorial & Production

Printed in the United States of America.

Contents

Introduction

As a medical educator, I have more than 20 years of teaching experience for pathophysiology. For my career, I have the opportunity for knowing and training many students. It is such a rewarding experience to guide students and witness them to succeed. On the other hand, some students did have troubles to figure out how to study the pathophysiology effectively. I believe a right tool can be developed to help all students who want to lay a solid foundation for studying medicine today. This is the motivation for me to work on this book.

How the Book is Organized

This book has 36 cases covering all the organ systems of pathophysiology. After a systemic study, the students can be trained to think independently, be a problem-solver, and/or become a great team player. The 36 cases are organized into 36 individual chapters, which has the content organized in the following order:

1. a table that consists of the acronym OLD CARTS (onset, location, duration, Characteristics, alleviating/aggravating factors, timing, and severity);
2. A brief introduction about the patient is presented including medical history, social history, family history, and other relevant information;
3. Findings from physical examination(s) and lab tests;
4. A list of possible differential diagnoses;
5. Diagnostic tests need to be ordered;
6. Treatment plan;
7. Prognosis

The book also has one appendix, which has detailed information on all current diagnostic procedures and equipment. Students can get familiar with them all at once before working on the chapters. I usually seek students for their feedback on which diagnostic procedure or equipment they have not heard or known, which would be a good starting point before diving into individual chapters (cases).

Author's Note to the Audience

To deliver a professional training experience, this book is written in scientific language with using medical terminology. The potential audience include undergraduate students (mainly juniors or seniors), professional students who are studying medicine in different school settings/specialty areas (allied health, dentistry, medicine, nursing, occupational therapy, osteopathic medicine, optometry, and physical therapy).

For educators, this book can be a useful tool for doing problem-based learning, team-based learning, or traditional teaching. Each case can be discussed in the classroom in different formats or assigned as supplemental readings. For working on an organ system, there are a few cases to choose. Depending on the time, you can decide how many cases you want the students to accomplish and in what format (classroom discussion, group assignment, individual reflection, etc.).

For students, this is the right tool for you to learn pathophysiology. I look forward to hearing your feedback for me to revise and improve the book to meet the needs. The old saying is true here: "Roma was not built in one day". But who we are tomorrow begins with what we do today.

Finally, I want to dedicate this book to my family for their endless support. It is they who always give me inspiration and encouragement, which motivate me and get my goals achieved in a timely manner.

Chapter 1

Nervous System: Case 1

Onset	The patient is a 58-year-old woman presenting with sudden onset of left facial drooping and left-sided weakness occurring at 11:50 a.m. August 2nd, 2023.
Location	• M2 branch (occlusion) • Brain (right frontal ischemic infarct) • Occlusion is consistent with cardioembolic because of newly found atrial flutter
Duration	Date of Admission: 8/2/2023 Date of Discharge: 8/5/2023 The symptoms had been present from August 2nd and were relieved on August 5th.
Characteristic	General left-sided weakness, plus left-sided facial droop
Alleviating Factors	Tissue plasminogen activator (tPA) administered shortly after onset
Aggravating Factors	
Timing	• Left-sided facial drooping subsided fully within 48 hours of onset • Overall left-sided drooping lasted 5 days • Spasticity in left arm remains
Severity	The patient came in scoring a 15 on the NIHSS (National Institutes of Health Stroke Scale), then improved on repeat NIHSS to a score of 5.

The NIHSS is a systemic, quantitative assessment tool for measuring stroke-related neurological deficit. The maximal score is 42 and the minimal score is 0. It is a tool used to objectively quantify the impairment due to a stroke. The tool assesses 11 specific abilities: level of consciousness (LOC), horizontal eye movement, visual field test, facial palsy, motor arm, motor leg, limb ataxia, sensory, language, speech, extinction, and inattention.

Score	Stroke Severity
0	No stroke symptoms
1–4	Minor stroke
5–15	Moderate stroke
16–20	Moderate to severe stroke
21–42	Severe stroke

Physical Examination

Neuro:	• Speech: dysarthric but spontaneous and fluent • Right gaze preference but able to cross midline • Asymmetrical left-sided mouth droop • Decreased sensation in left face and arm • Spasticity of left lower arm • Unable to lift left upper extremities (LUE) and has difficulty moving left lower extremities (LLE)
Overall examination:	• Head is atraumatic and normocephalic • Eyes: Pupils are equal, round, reactive to light, and able to accommodate • The trachea is midline and there is no presence of jugular vein distention • Air is moving well, and breaths sounds are symmetrical • Heart shows regular rate and rhythm • Gastrointestinal examination showed soft GI, not distended, normal bowel sounds, and non-tender • Extremities showed adequate distal perfusion and 2+ pulses (slightly more diminished) throughout • Skin examination: intact, warm and dry, and shows no abnormalities • Preserved ejection fraction • Hypertensive • Hyperlipidemia

Step 1: What are possible diagnoses (3–5)?

1. Hemorrhagic stroke
2. Ischemic stroke
3. Viral infection

Step 2: Based on the medical history, which diagnostic tests should you order?

Lab on 08/04/2023

Component		Normal Range
Sodium	143	135–145 mEq/L
Potassium	3.5	3.6–5.2 mmol/L
Chloride	110	96–106 mEq/L
BUN	11	5–20 mg/dL
Creatinine (blood)	0.76	0.6–1.2 mg/dL
Glucose (blood)	111	70–100 mg/dL(fasting)
Calcium	8.6	8.6–10.3 mg/dL
WBC	8.9	4.5–11 x 10^9/L
Hemoglobin	12.3	12–15.5 g/dL (female); 13.5–17.5 g/dL (male)
Hematocrit	38	36–48 (female); 40–54 (male)
Platelets	234	150–450 x 10^9/L

Diagnostic Tests

Head/neck computed tomography Angiography (CTA) with perfusion	• Occlusion of right M2 branch • Distal branches suggest good reconstitution • No evidence of high-grade stenosis, hemorrhage, or acute finding in cervical carotid or vertebral arteries
Dual energy CT of head	No evidence of acute intracranial hemorrhage
Brain MRI	Showed acute right frontal ischemic infarct
Transthoracic Echocardiogram (TTE)	• Mild left atrial enlargement • Mild aortic insufficiency • Grade 3 diastolic dysfunction
EKG	Atrial flutter diagnosed and determined to be etiological cause

Step 3: Based on the information on the patient presentation, diagnostic tests, and medical history, what is your decision regarding treating the patient? Why?

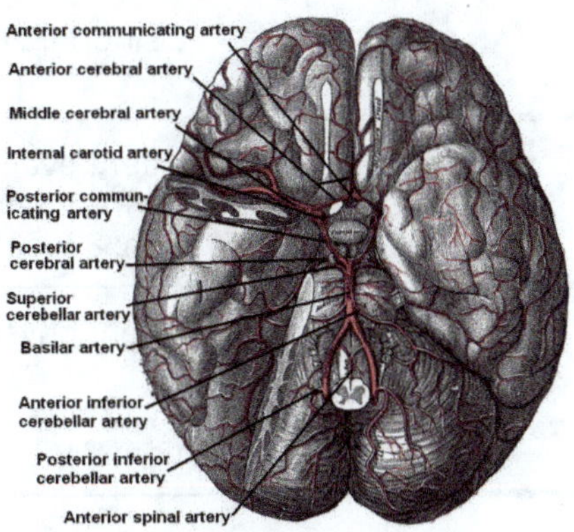

Figure 1.1 Brain Blood Supply

Treatment Plan

Medication	New medications: • Apixaban 5 mg: anticoagulant • 1 tablet by mouth 2x daily For atrial fibrillation/atrial flutter • Atorvastatin80 mg: • 1 tablet by mouth daily Modified Medications: • Atenolol 25 mg: • 1 tablet by mouth every12 hours Medication continuations: • Aspirin 81mg: • 1 tablet by mouth every night Transitioned to apixaban (Eliquis) on 8/7/2023 • Cetirizine 10mg: • 1 tablet by mouth daily • Multivitamin: • 1 capsule by mouth daily. Stopped medications: • Lisinopril 20 mg
Occupational Therapy	Outpatient evaluation and treatment Weekly frequency: 3 Duration: 8 weeks
Physical Therapy	Outpatient physical therapy evaluation and treatment Weekly frequency: 3 Duration: 8 weeks

Step 4: What are the risk factors for ischemic stroke?

1. Atrial flutter
2. Hypertension
3. Hyperlipidemia
4. Heart failure with preserved ejection fraction

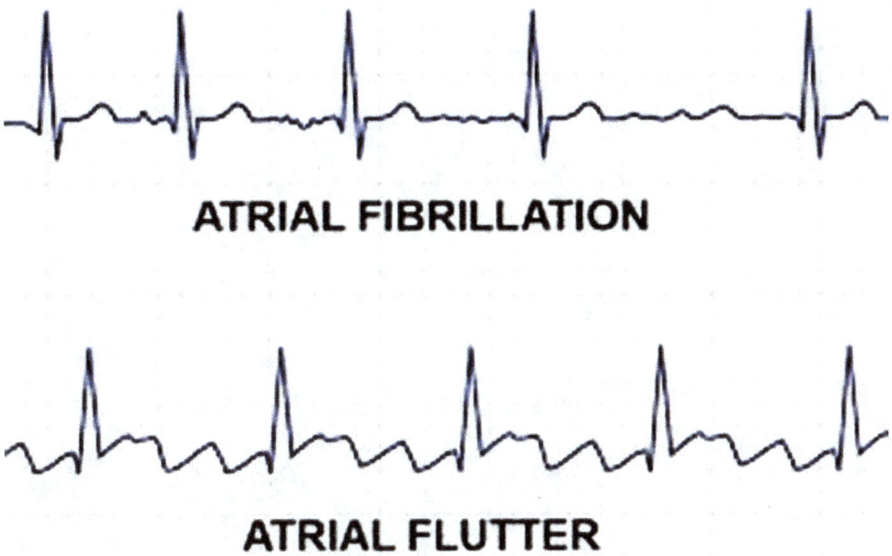

Figure 1.2 ECGs for Atrial Fibrillation and Atrial Flutter

Follow-Up

1. Hospital follow-up to neurology
2. Hospital follow-up to sleep medicine
3. Hospital follow-up to cardiology
4. Transthoracic echo (TTE) completed with or without contrast per protocol with bubble study

Step 5: What have you learned from this case?

1. How does one differentiate between hemorrhagic and ischemic strokes?

2. What is the normal procedure for treating an ischemic stroke?

Image Credits:

Fig. 1.1: Henry Gray and Wikid77, https://commons.wikimedia.org/wiki/File:Arteries_beneath_brain_Gray_closer.jpg, 1918.

Fig. 1.2: Copyright © 2023 by IRHTO (CC BY-ND 4.0) at https://irhto.com/cardiology/atrial-fibrillation-andflutter/.

Chapter 2

Digestive System: Case 1

Onset	The patient is a 48-year-old Asian male who presented for a regular dental check at 1:30 p.m. on July 12th, 2023.
Location	Gums
Duration	Bleed when brushing teeth before bedtime
Characteristic	Bleed from time to time when brushing teeth
Alleviating Factors	None
Aggravating Factors	None
Timing	Stop after brushing the teeth
Severity	Slight

Blood pressure: 116/90 mm Hg; Pulse: 90 beats per minute; Temperature: 98° F; Respiratory rate: 16/minute

Physical Examination	• Head is atraumatic and normocephalic • Eyes: Pupils are equal, round, reactive to light, and able to accommodate • Trachea is midline, and there is no presence of jugular vein distention • Air is movingwell, and breaths sounds are symmetrical • Heart shows regular rate and rhythm. • Gastrointestinal examination showed soft GI, notdistended, normal bowel sounds, and non-tender • Extremities showed adequate distal perfusion. • Skin examination shows no abnormalities; intact, warm, and dry

Social History: One or two beers/week; does not smoke.

Medical History

- Left lower wisdom tooth was extracted in December 2016
- Abdominal hernia on the right side was surgically repaired (patched) in September 2012
- Has not had a dental visit in the past 5 years

Diagnostic Tests	Dental X-ray

Step 1: What are possible diagnoses (3–5)?

1. Periodontal disease
2. Vitamin C deficiency
3. Hemophilia

Step 2: Based on the medical history, what diagnostic tests should you order?

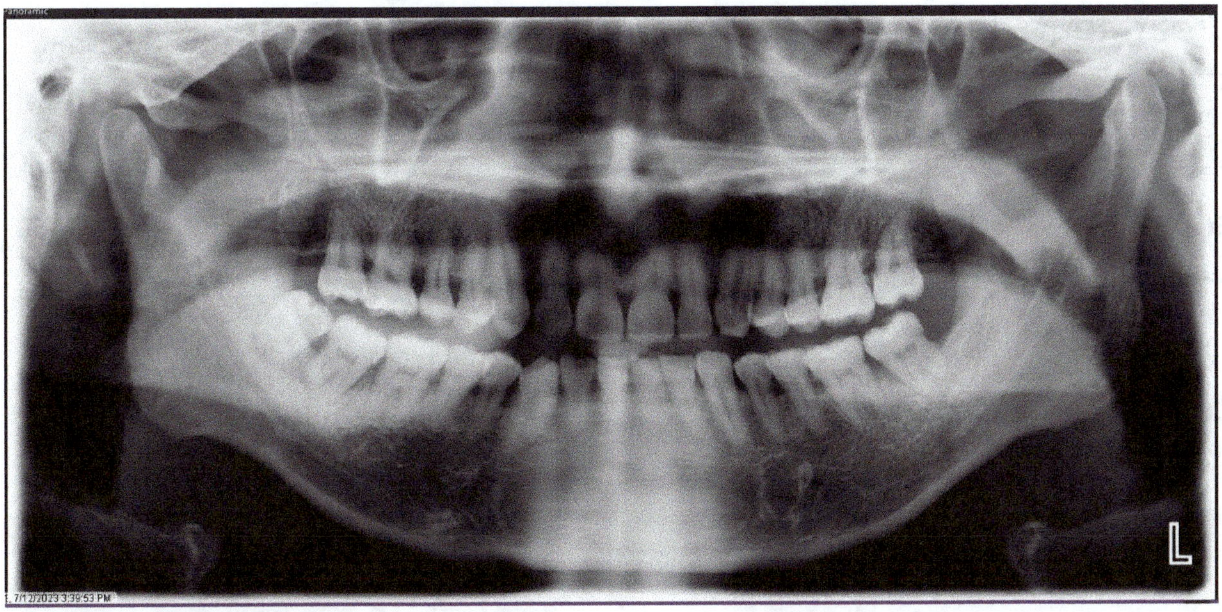

Figure 2.1a Dental X-Ray

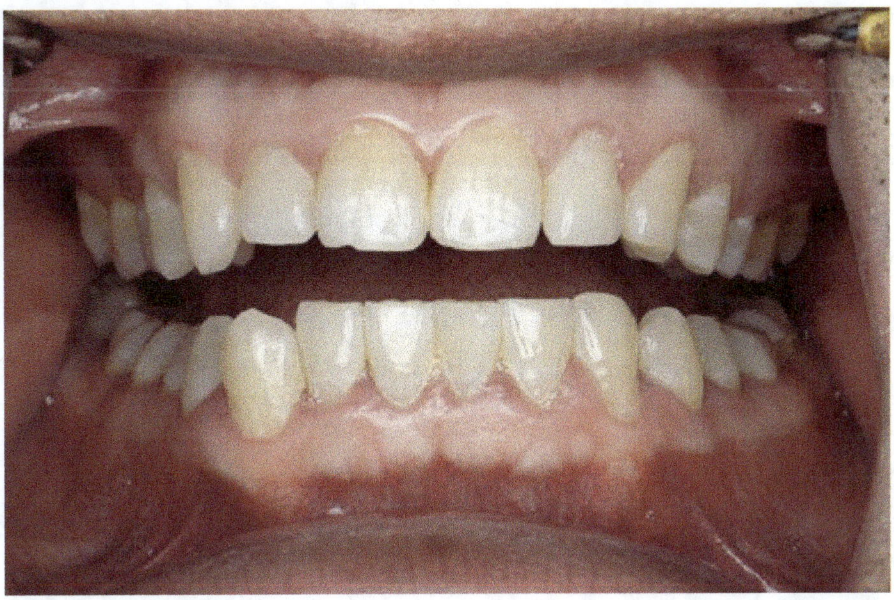

Figure 2.1b Dental Picture

Step 3: Based on the information on the patient presentation, diagnostic tests, medical history, what is your decision regarding treating the patient? Why?

Treatment Plan

Deep cleaning to remove the calculus Follow up in two weeks	Brush twice a day and use dental floss

Step 4: What are the risk factors for getting periodontal disease?

1. Poor oral hygiene
2. Smoking
3. Lack of regular dental care

Step 5: What have you learned from this case?

1. How does one prevent the development of periodontal disease?

Chapter 3

Endocrine System: Case 1

Onset	The patient is a 21-year-old White female. She has abdominal pain beginning four years after menarche.
Location	Lower central abdomen
Duration	Started at age 16 and has lasted approximately five years
Characteristic	Varying dull and cramping pain; pain radiates toward the hips
Alleviating Factors	Heating pad, yoga, Advil, cooling and heating therapies
Aggravating Factors	Exercise in hot weather, menstruation
Timing	Constant pain
Severity	Pain is 4/10 but can get to 6–7/10

HOMA-IR stands for Homeostatic Model Assessment for Insulin Resistance. It is calculated by multiplying fasting plasma insulin (FPI) in the unit of microU/L by fasting plasma glucose (FPG) in the unit of nmol/L, then dividing by 22.5. A normal HOMA-IR should be less than 2.5.

Physical Examination

- Body weight is about 200 lbs.; body mass index (BMI) ≥ 34
- Alopecia (diffuse non-scarring type)
- Acne
- Irregular menstrual cycle (cycle length can be as along as 50 days or as short as 12 days)
- Moon face
- Oligomenorrhea

Step 1: What are possible diagnoses (3–5)?

1. Polycystic ovary syndrome
2. Hypothyroidism
3. Cushing syndrome/disease
4. Pituitary adenoma

Step 2: Based on the medical history, what diagnostic tests should you order?

Step 3: Based on the information on the patient presentation, diagnostic tests, medical history, what is your decision regarding treating the patient? Why?

Treatment Plan

Clomifene can stimulate ovulation and regular monthly menstruation. It is the first-line treatment for women with PCOS who are trying to get pregnant. If unsuccessful in stimulating ovulation, **metformin** is usually recommended.	Metformin is often used to treat type 2 diabetes. It can also aid in lowering insulin and blood glucose levels in patients with PCOS.
Oral contraceptive can be used to treat alopecia and hirsutism. • Eflornithine can be used to slow the growth of unwanted hair and may be used with a hair removal product.	Anti-androgens may be offered to combat excessive hair growth. • Spironolactone is an androgen receptor antagonist that can stop dihydrotestosterone (DHT) expression by competing with testosterone or DHT to bind with their receptors. • Finasteride is a 5-alpha reductase inhibitor that can inhibit the conversion from testosterone to DHT.
Control BMI and body weight. Laparoscopic ovarian drilling to rebalance and improve ovarian function.	

Step 4: What are the risk factors for getting PCOS?

Genetic (inheritance)

Follow-Up Measures	• HOMA-IR • Insulin: 45 microU/mL; blood glucose: 80 mg/dL; insulin resistance: 1; Beta cell function: 594.41%; Insulin sensitivity: 9.97% • Free testosterone: 0 pg/mL (normal range: 0–8 pg/mL) • Total testosterone: 22.9 ng/dL (normal range: 0.5–118 ng/dL) • DHEA-S: 349 µg/dL (normal range: 35–430 µg/dL) • LH: ≤ 0.07 international units (IU)/L • FSH: ≤ 0.3 IU/L

The pancreas likely will not be able to keep up with the need in the future (burnt out).

Step 5: What have you learned from this case?

There are different types of PCOS: inflammatory, post pill, adrenal, and insulin resistant. What is insulin-resistant PCOS?

Insulin-resistant PCOS is a common type of PCOS. Patients who have this type of PCOS are insulin resistant, meaning that their bodies can make insulin but cannot use it efficiently. Excessive insulin can drive the overproduction of ovarian androgen. The common manifestations are diabetes, heart disease, infertility, menstrual abnormalities, and overweightness.

Chapter 4

Reproductive System: Case 1

Onset	A hard, irregular lump was noticed by the patient in January 2021 when she was conducting routine self-breast examination.
Location	Right breast around 7 o'clock position
Duration	The mass exists since January 2021
Characteristic	The mass is 1.6 cm in diameter, hard, painless, and irregular. Not tender.
Alleviating Factors	None
Aggravating Factors	None
Timing	No pain
Severity	n/a

Physical Examination

- A mass was found by the patient when she conducted routine self-breast exam in January 2021.
- The mass is hard, irregular, and not painful.
- The mass is in the right breast at 7 o'clock position.
- Patient denies any soreness, fever.
- No redness or swelling were seen in the local area.

Step 1: What are possible diagnoses (3–5)?

1. Breast cancer
2. Fibroadenoma
3. Cysts

Step 2: Based on the medical history, what diagnostic tests should you order?

Bilateral Mammogram: A 1.6cm spiculated mass was found in the lower right breast at the 7 o'clock position with a few associated amorphous microcalcifications.

Ultrasound: Right breast ultrasound showed a mixed hyper- and hypo-echoic solid mass measuring 1.6 x 1.9 x 0.8 cm. Margins are indistinct. There is no internal blood flow. The ultrasound also demonstrated two smooth round anechoic masses consistent with simple cysts. "Hyperechoic" means lots of echoes and refers to areas that appear light gray on ultrasound. Cysts filled with air or fluid are usually hyperechoic and rarely cancerous. They are usually not as dense as hypoechoic masses. "Hypoechoic" means not many echoes and refers to areas that appear dark gray because they do not send back a lot of sound waves. Solid masses of dense tissue are hypoechoic and can be cancerous.

Biopsy: A right breast biopsy was performed on the mass. The pathology confirmed 1.9 cm right breast ductal carcinoma in situ (DCIS) with ductal and lobular features. Four lymph nodes were cancer negative. It is Stage 1 breast cancer. ER (+++), Her2 equivocal. Margins are negative with the closest invasive at 4 mm. Left breast was negative for invasive or in situ carcinoma.

Invasive ductal carcinoma is the most common type of breast cancer. "Ductal" means the cancer started in the milk ducts. Ductal carcinoma in situ (DCIS), also called intraductal carcinoma, is a pre-invasive breast cancer. The cells lining the ducts have changed to cancerous, but they have not broken the wall of the ducts and spread into the surround breast tissue.

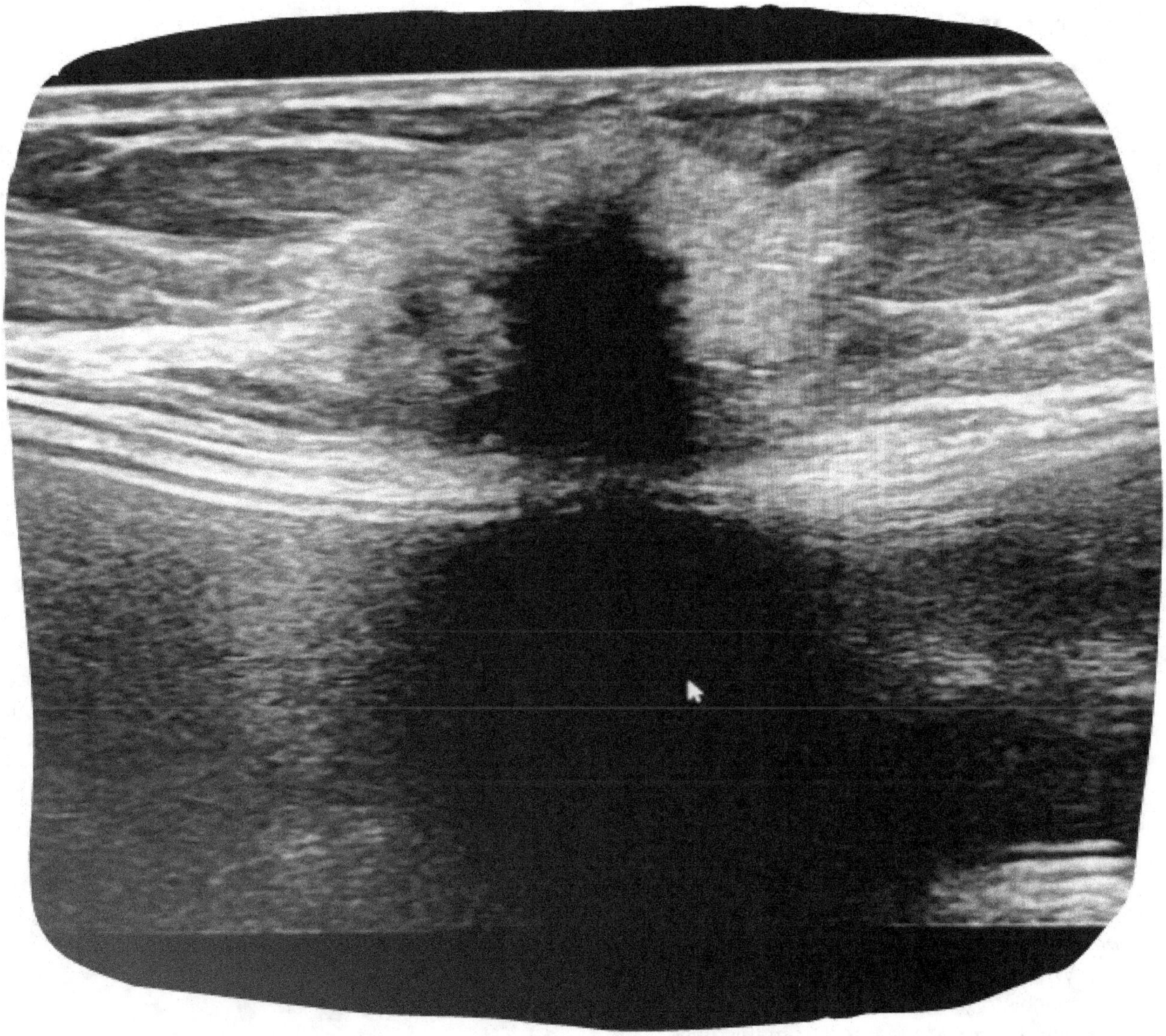

Figure 4.1 Breast Ultrasound

Step 3: Based on the information on the patient presentation, diagnostic tests, and medical history, what is your decision regarding treating the patient? Why?

Treatment Plan

• Bilateral mastectomy with latissimus flap and expanders • Reconstruction was done in April 2021	• After surgery, tramadol is used for managing pain. Antibiotics and blood thinners were used as well.
• Arm exercises such as shoulder shrugs and circles help prevent scar tissue formation. • Deep breathing • Walking • No lifting objects heavier than 5 pounds for 6 weeks post op. • Refrained from lifting arms over the head for at least one week.	• Medications: tamoxifen • No chemotherapy or radiation therapy • No diet recommendation

Mastectomy is the first treatment for many types of breast cancer such as DCIS, stage 1 or 2 breast cancer, Paget's disease of the breast, and locally recurrent breast cancer. In addition, mastectomy can be done after chemo for stage 3 breast cancer or inflammatory breast cancer.

Double mastectomy with latissimus flap reconstruction and tissue expanders: 1) the procedure lasted about 8 hours; 2) all breast tissues were removed; 3) latissimus muscle was tunneled under the arm to the breast area, and a pocket was created for the tissue expanders to be placed beneath; 4) four surgical drains were inserted in the breast area to prevent fluid accumulation (tubes carry fluid out of the body to an attached soft plastic bag); 4) sentinel node biopsy and removal of 1–5 lymph nodes, into which the cancer drains. The nodes were found using a radioactive tracer and dye injected on the day of surgery. Lymph nodes were negative for cancer.

Reconstruction: 1) Tissue expanders were removed and replaced with the permanent silicone implants; 2) Nipple reconstruction and additional fat grafting (used to fill imperfections and thicken the layer of tissue between an implant and the skin) were also performed to improve the natural look of the breast.

Step 4: What are the risk factors for getting breast cancer?

Family history

Step 5: What have you learned from this case?

Diagnosis and treatment of breast cancer

Chapter 5

Circulatory System: Case 1

Onset	The patient is a 60-year-old Asian female complaining of dyspnea and severe chest pain.
Location	Upper chest
Duration	Started to feel fatigue, dyspnea, and chest pain after returning from a trip in March 2023
Characteristic	Sharp and constant pain in the chest
Alleviating Factors	none
Aggravating Factors	
Timing	Constant pain
Severity	Pain is 7/10

Social history: Does not smoke or drink; divorced; one son

Medical history: A cholecystectomy was done when the patient was 40 years old.

Step 1: What are possible diagnoses (3–5)?

1. Cancer
2. Pericardial effusion
3. Tuberculosis
4. COVID-19

Step 2: Based on the medical history, what diagnostic tests should you order?

CT (3-27-2023)

The CT shows pericardial effusion and inflammation around lower lobes of both lungs. No plural effusion or plural membrane thickness; dilation of common hepatic duct; increased density of soft tissue in the mediastinum and could not be distinct from surrounding tissue.

Patient lost more than 25 pounds in about two months, had night sweats, and did not sleep well. Low fever in a random pattern each day. No medication (NSAID) is effective for the fever.

PET-CT (5-3-2023)

Metabolically active soft tissue areas in pericardium and mediastinum; pericardial effusion; active lymph nodes can be seen in bilateral cervical II-III areas and left cervical IV area; inflammation in the left lung and left plural effusion; liver cyst

Blood lab test (5-16-2023)

Monocyte percentage: 14.5% (3%–10%)

C-reactive protein: 39.83 (0–5) mg/L

Interleukin-6: 19.8 (0–7) pg/mL

Calcitonin: 0.048 (0–0.046) ng/mL

Immunohistochemistry (needle biopsy from mediastinal lymph node 6-29-2023)

CK(-); Vimentin (-); LCA (+); CD5(+); CD117 (-); TdT (-); TIF-1 (-); P40 (-); CD20 (+); CgA (-); Syn (-); CD56 (-); CD1A (-), CD3 (-); PAX-5 (+); Ki-67 (90%+)

Diagnosis: Non-Hodgkin's lymphoma (NHL): diffuse large B-cell lymphoma (DLBCL)

Step 3: Based on the patient presentation, diagnostic tests, and medical history, what is your decision regarding treating the patient? Why?

CD40 is a molecule expressed on the cell surface of lymphoma cells, and antibodies such as rituximab target this molecule. The most commonly used chemotherapy regimen is R CHOP (rituximab, cyclophosphamide, doxorubicin, vincristine, and prednisone); it is usually given in 21-day cycles. Sometimes etoposide is added to the R CHOP regimen.

Step 4: What are the risk factors for getting DLBCL?

1. Radiation exposure
2. Age
3. Family history
4. Virus exposure (flu)

Step 5: What have you learned from this case?

Diffuse large B-cell lymphoma (DLBCL) is the most common type of non-Hodgkin lymphoma (NHL), and it is malignant. The incidence generally increases with age, with most patients being over the age of 60 at diagnosis. Primary mediastinal B-cell lymphoma is a subtype of DLBCL.

Diagnosis and treatment of DLBCL.

Is CART effective?

Chapter 6

Respiratory System: Case 1

Onset	The patient is a 21-year-old White female who complains of pain and malaise for about 6 days.
Location	Inflamed tonsils with white exudate, muscle aches, and fatigue
Duration	Pain and malaise lasted 6 days
Characteristic	Constant but worse in the mornings, slowly getting worse from the onset
Alleviating Factors	Taking ibuprofen every 6 hours provides some relief
Aggravating Factors	Painful swallowing, extreme fatigue with activities
Timing	Constant pain
Severity	Pain is 4/10

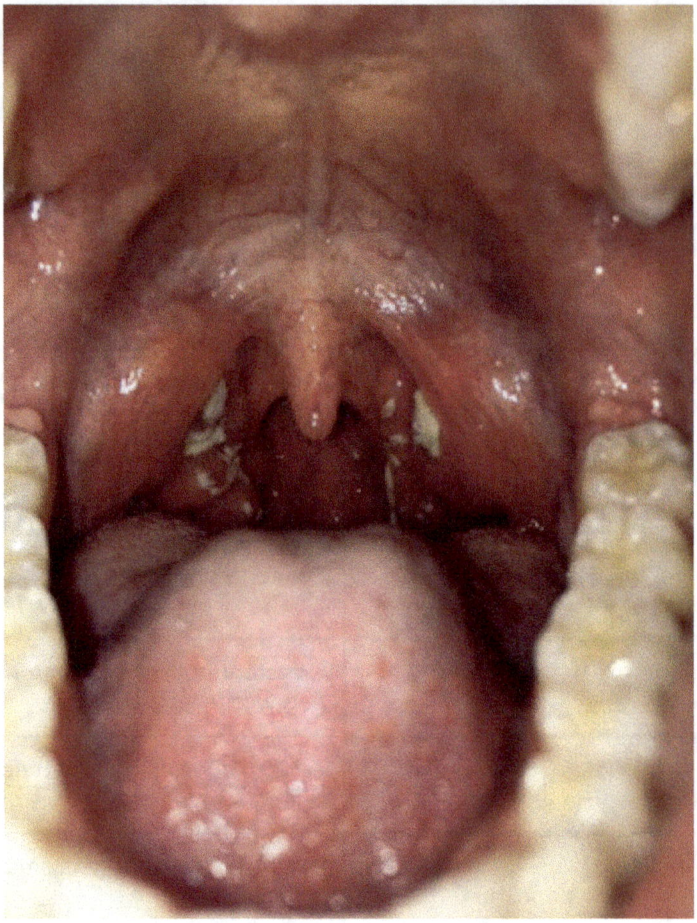

Figure 6.1 Throat and Oral Cavity Picture

On September 5th, 2023, the patient noticed a sore throat, muscle aches, and fatigue.

Physical Examination

- No pharyngeal erythema, no tonsillar enlargement or exudate. No cervical lymphadenopathy was found.
- Heart: Regular heart rate and rhythm. No murmur.
- Lungs: clear
- Skin: no rash

The following tests are negative (flu, strep, and COVID-19). Treatment plan included hydration, rest, and Ibuprofen: nonsteroid anti-inflammatory drugs (NSAIDs).

Medical History: On September 8th, 2023, the patient complained of recurring high fevers, extreme fatigue, and muscle pain (6/10). Physical examination indicated an elevated heart rate, tonsillar erythema, white tonsillar exudate, and an elevated temperature. Vital signs were 110 (HR), 99% (SaO2), 115/79 mmHg (BP), and 101.4oF (temperature). Strep test was negative and Monospot test was positive. Treatment plan was adjusted to include prednisone (10 mg), NSAIDs, rest, hydration, and lifestyle modifications (reduce movement) to reduce the risk of splenic rupture within one month. Stop consumption of caffeine and alcohol.

Constant vomiting and nausea started the night of September 10th, 2023, accompanied by a sore throat and swallowing pain (6–7/10). Muscle pain and fatigue had gotten worse. Physical examination showed a mild distension of abdomen. Nontoxic appearance and no acute distress. The neck is supple and no thyromegaly. Cervical adenopathy was seen. Regular heart rate and rhythm. Lungs are clear to auscultation bilaterally. No edema was seen in extremities. Rapid strep test is used to rule out secondary strep infection.

Step 1: What are possible diagnoses (3–5)?

1. Mononucleosis
2. Strep throat
3. Flu
4. COVID-19

Step 2: Based on the medical history, what diagnostic tests should you order?

Lab Results

Test	Result	Flags	Reference Range
Glucose	87		65–99 mg/dL
Urea nitrogen	8		7–25 mg/dL
Creatinine	0.7		0.5–0.96 mg/dL
EGFR	126		> or = 60 mL/min/ 1.73m2
BUN/Creatinine ratio	normal		6–22 (calculation)
Sodium	139		135–146 mmol/L
Potassium	4.1		3.5–5.3 mmol/L
Chloride	104		98–110 mmol/L
Carbon Dioxide	24		20–32 mmol/L
Protein (total)	6.8		6.1–8.1 g/dL
Albumin	4		3.6–5.1 g/dL
Globulin	2.8		1.9–3.7 g/dL (calculation)
Albumin/Globulin Ratio	1.4		1.0–2.5 (calculation)
Bilirubin (total)	0.7		0.2–1.2 mg/dL
Alkaline Phosphatase	254	H	31–125 U/L
AST	175	H	10–30 U/L
ALT	339	H	6–29 U/L
White Blood Cell Count	12.7	H	3.8–10.8 *1000/uL
Red Blood Cell Count	4.12		3.8–5.1 million/uL
Hemoglobin	12.5		11.7–15.5 g/dL
Hematocrit	37.1		35%–45%

Test	Result	Flags	Reference Range
MCV	90		80–100 fL
MCH	30.3		27–33 pg
MCHC	33.7		32–36 g/dL
RDW	13.4		11%–15%
Platelet Count	196		140–400*1000/uL
MPV	9.6		7.5–12.5 fL
Absolute Neutrophils	7112		1500–7800 cells/uL
Absolute Lymphocytes	3810		850–3900 cells/uL
Absolute Reactive Lymphocytes	508	H	0
Absolute Monocytes	1143	H	200–950 cells/uL
Absolute Eosinophils	127		15–500 cells/uL
Absolute Basophils	0		0–200 cells/uL
Neutrophils	56		%
Lymphocytes	30		%
Reactive Lymphocytes	4		0%–10%
Monocytes	9		%
Eosinophils	1		%
Basophils	0		%

Step 3: Based on the patient presentation, diagnostic tests, and medical history, what is your decision regarding treating the patient? Why?

Blood tests (complete blood count [CBC] and comprehensive metabolic panel [CMP]) were performed. The treatment plan included hydration, Zofran (ondansetron 4 mg/every 6–8 hours, oral tablet) for nausea, and monitoring for secondary strep infection. Steroids (dexamethasone sodium phosphate 4 mg IM) were used for symptoms. Sticking to ibuprofen over acetaminophen was prescribed due to elevated liver enzymes associated with mononucleosis.

Good nutrition is recommended.

Step 4: What are the risk factors for having mononucleosis?

Age

Step 5: What have you learned from this case?

Mononucleosis is a contagious infection caused by Epstein–Barr virus (EBV). It typically spreads through direct contact and is commonly transmitted through saliva. EBV targets the salivary glands and oropharyngeal epithelium. It infects local lymphoid tissue and B cells. Then the infection spreads through the lymphatic system. The liver and spleen can be affected as well.

EBV belongs to the Herpesviridae family. It contains a linear, double-stranded DNA molecule. Signs and symptoms include fever, fatigue, malaise, headache, muscle ache/weakness, swollen lymphoid tissue, inflamed tonsils with purulent white patches, and enlargement of the spleen and/or liver.

Chapter 7

Musculoskeletal System: Case 1

Onset	A 20-year-old White female presents with polyarthralgia, primarily affecting her wrists and hands for 6 months prior to visit (December 2021).
Location	Bilateral wrists, hands, lower back, and toes
Duration	6 months
Characteristic	Stiffness/aches are worse in the morning and improve throughout the day; tightness and stiffness in her back as well; Raynaud's discoloration of fingers and toes; fatigue
Alleviating Factors	NSAIDs, use of heating pad on hands helps reduce the pain,
Aggravating Factors	Repetitive joint use
Timing	Pain is persistent and worse in the morning; stiffness is intermittent and worse upon waking
Severity	Pain is 7/10

Social History: non-smoker

Past Medical History: asthma, food, and environmental allergies

Vital Signs: 141/89 mm Hg (BP), 77 beats per minute (HR), 96% (SaO2), 97.9°F (temperature)

Body Weight: 150 lbs.

The patient has polyarthralgia in bilateral wrists, hands, lower back, and toes. More pain was felt in wrists, thumbs, and index fingers. The pain is radiating through the hand joints but not in other joints of the body. The lower back had localized pain and stiffness. No pain was found with feet, but Raynaud's discoloration was seen in both fingers and toes. Symptoms began gradually but became more noticeable and persistent with time. No known injury or cause predated the onset of symptoms.

Stiffness and pain were significantly worse in the mornings after waking, lasting for approximately one to two hours before becoming dull. All symptoms occurred every day but were more intense on some days than others. Symptoms were relieved midday and recurred later in the day with use of hands.

Pain and stillness interfere with daily use and activities such as writing, typing, and fine motor movements involving the hands.

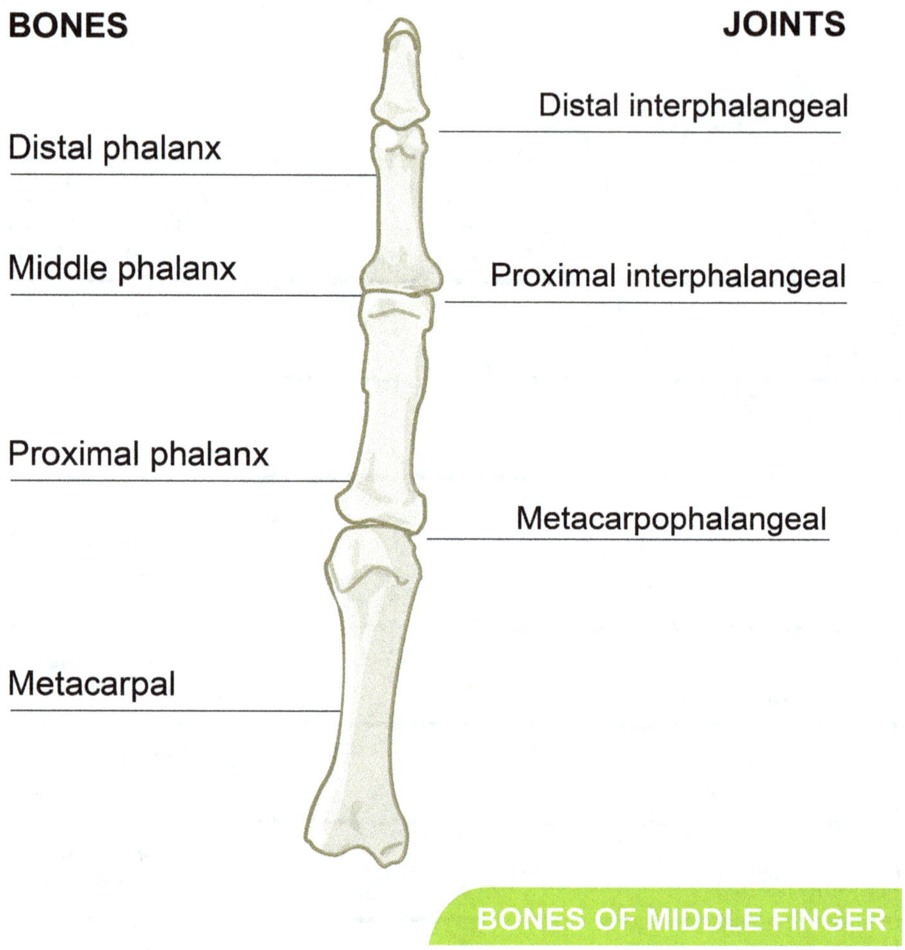

Figure 7.1 Finger Joints

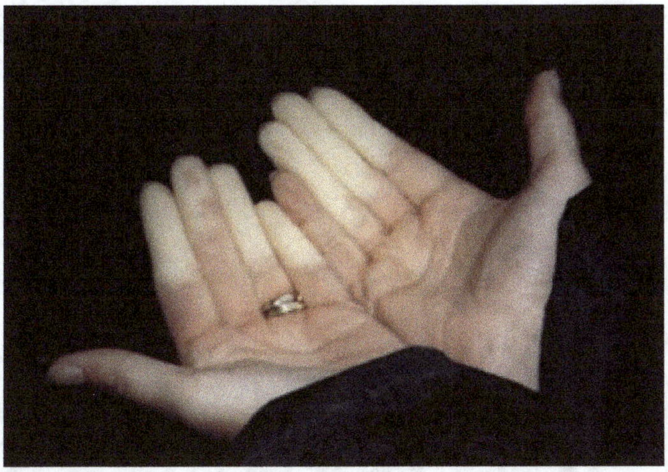

Figure 7.2 Raynaud's Discoloration

Step 1: What are possible diagnoses?

1. Early rheumatoid arthritis
2. Seronegative spondyloarthropathy
3. Systemic lupus erythematosus

Polyarthralgia was confirmed, and there was suspicion of small joint arthritis in her hands. Tenderness in bilateral second and third MCPs (metacarpophalangeal joint). Range of motion is normal. Right posterior SI (sacroiliac) joint is tender.

Step 2: Based on the medical history, what diagnostic tests should you order?

Serological tests:

1. ANA (antinuclear antibody) titer was 1:160, speckled. Speckled pattern correlates with antibody to nuclear antigens. It is found in many different diseases.

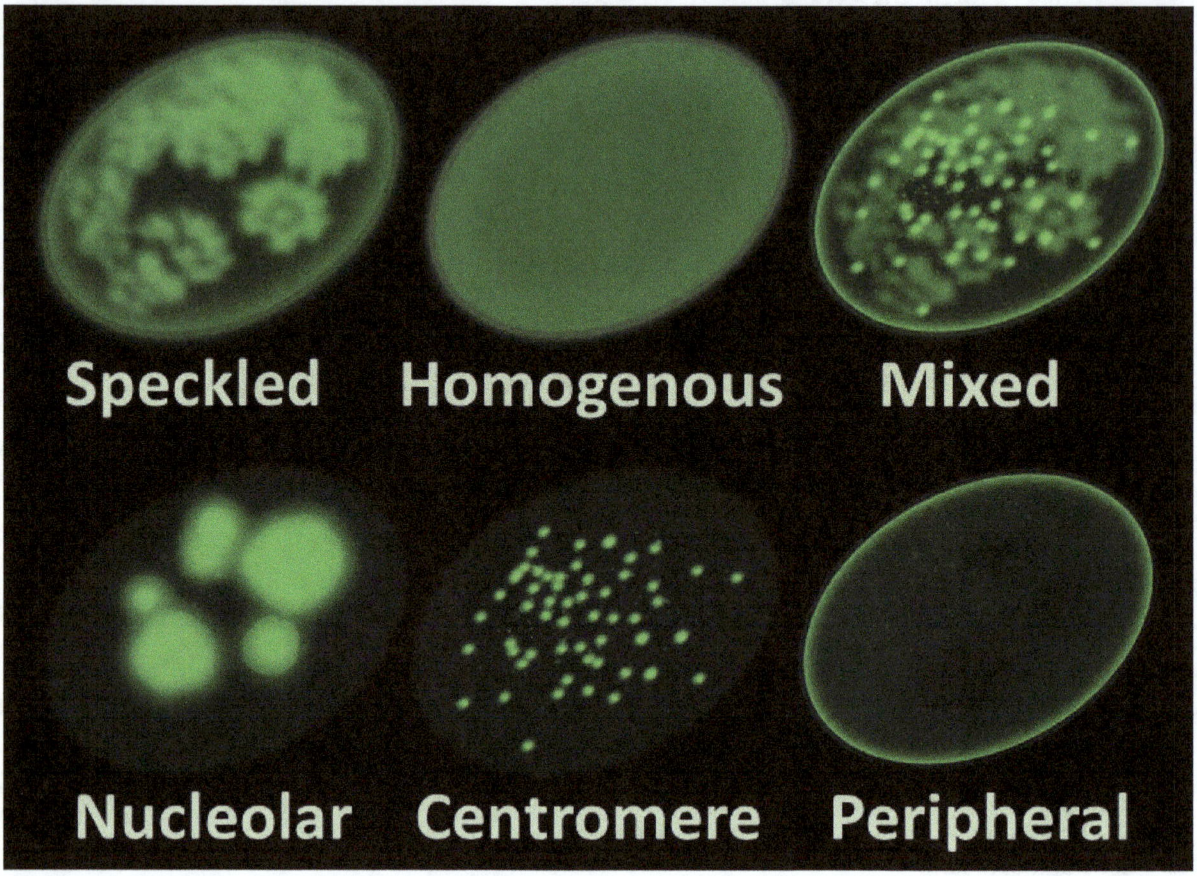

Figure 7.3 Fluorescent Antinuclear Antibody Test

- CRP: 6.64 mg/L with a normal range of 0–10.9 mg/L
- Rheumatoid factor (RF): 110 IU/mL with a normal range of 0–14 IU/mL
- Erythrocyte sedimentation rate (ESR): 11 mm/h with a normal range of 0–20 mm/h
- Anti-dsDNA: negative (systemic lupus erythematosus was ruled out).
- Anti-CCP (IgG): < 13 units with a normal range of 0–19 units
- Ultrasound of the hands to evaluate joint inflammation
- Mild synovial thickening of the second MCPs indicated mild synovitis.
- X-rays of the hands and feet to assess joint damage

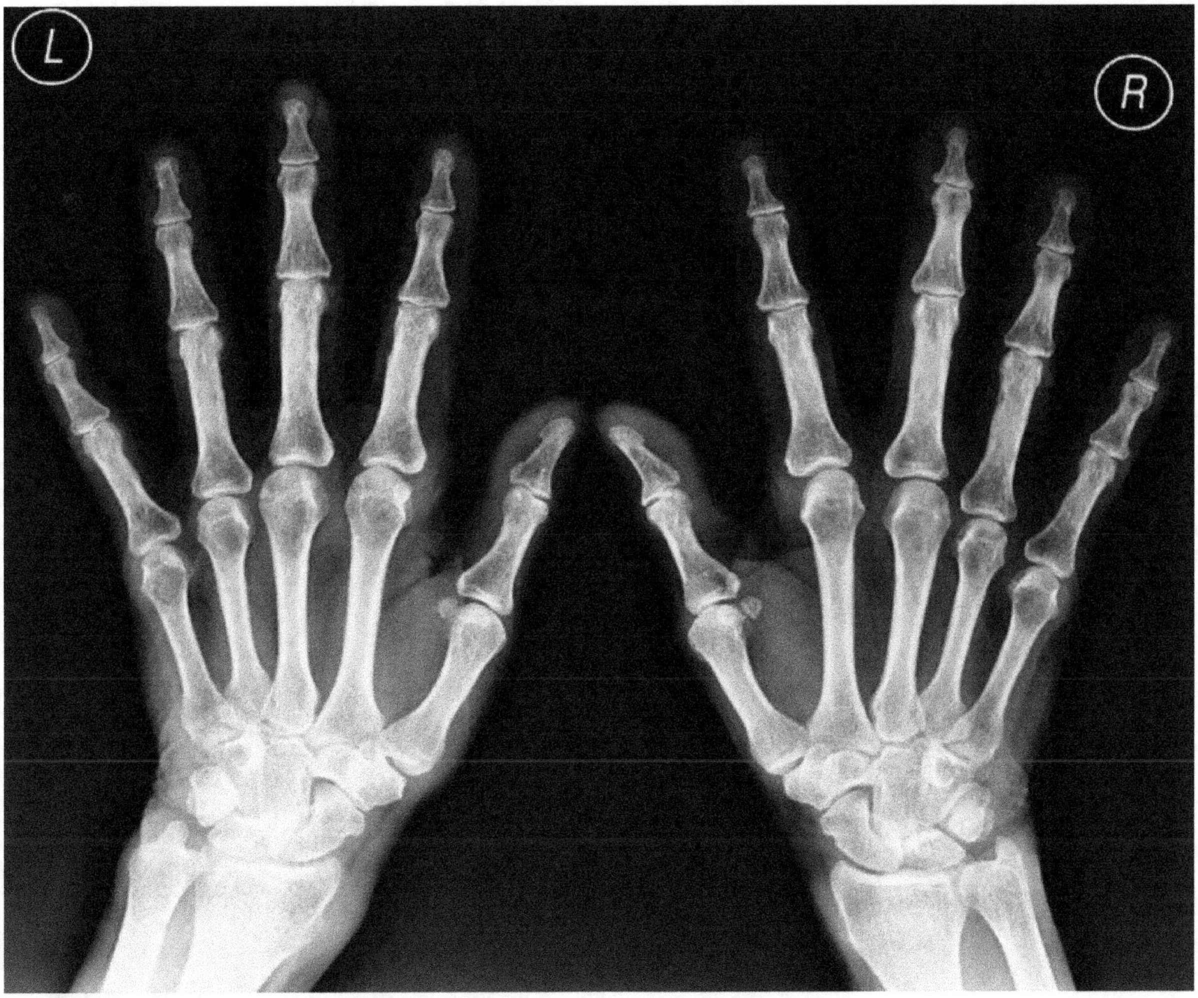

Figure 7.4 X-ray of the Hand Joints

No erosion was seen, joint spaces were well maintained, and the bone density was normal.

Differential diagnosis:

1. Early rheumatoid arthritis: joint pain, swollen joints, fatigue, positive ANA, positive RF
    - Does not support: positive ANA (speckled)
2. Seronegative spondyloarthropathy: inflammatory joint pain that improves with time/activities; back pain
    - Do not support: location of the joint pain, positive RF
3. Systemic lupus erythematosus: joint pain, swollen joints, fatigue, speckled ANA
    - Do not support: no malar rash, no weight loss, no photosensitivity

Diagnosis of Early Rheumatoid Arthritis

Rheumatoid arthritis is an autoimmune disorder that causes chronic systemic inflammation in the joints. This inflammation is caused by the immune system targeting and attacking healthy cells.

The pathophysiology includes

- Pannus formation
- Synovitis
- Erosion of cartilage
- Fibrosis
- Muscle atrophy
- Muscle spasms
- Joint/bone deformities

Systemic effects:

- Stiffness
- Impaired joint movement
- Finger/wrist inflammation
- Fatigue
- Anorexia
- Malaise
- Fever
- Iron deficiency
- Red, swollen joints

RA is usually seen more in women than men, but it can affect any age group. It has familial predisposition and can depend on a genetic factor, but it also can be linked to some viral infections.

Due to the age of the patient, RA is deemed to be in the early stages.

Treatment

No surgery recommended.

No diet recommendations.

15 mg Mobic (meloxicam) once daily. It is an NSAID used specifically for RA or osteoarthritis to reduce inflammation and pain.

Hydroxychloroquine 200 mg once daily

- Antimalarial and antirheumatic drug (disease-modifying antirheumatic drug [DMARD])
- Used to treat RA and SLE
- Immunosuppressive and immunomodulatory

Prognosis

1. Disease will continue to progress but there is a possible chance of natural remission.
2. Increased chance of early death (2x more likely to die than someone of same age without disease)
3. Possible future treatments:
4. Corticosteroid injections to relieve joint inflammation

5. Further use of DMARDs:
    - methotrexate
    - leflunomide
    - sulfasalazine

Image Credits

Chapter 8

Respiratory System: Case 2

Onset	A 23-year-old Black female was rushed to the emergency room with complaints of shortness of breath. She was coughing and sneezing uncontrollably.
Location	Upper chest
Duration	Symptoms began shortly after taking a single ibuprofen tablet.
Characteristic	Nasal polyps and rhinitis
Alleviating Factors	None
Aggravating Factors	
Timing	
Severity	

Past medical history: She suffered from childhood asthma that began around 8 months old and stopped around age 6.

Family history: Both her brother and her paternal grandmother have asthma.

Step 1: What are possible diagnoses (3–5)?

1. Asthma
2. Drug allergy
3. Foreign object aspiration

Step 2: Based on the medical history, what diagnostic tests should you order?

Chest X-Ray: to identify any foreign bodies in the airway and check for pneumonia.

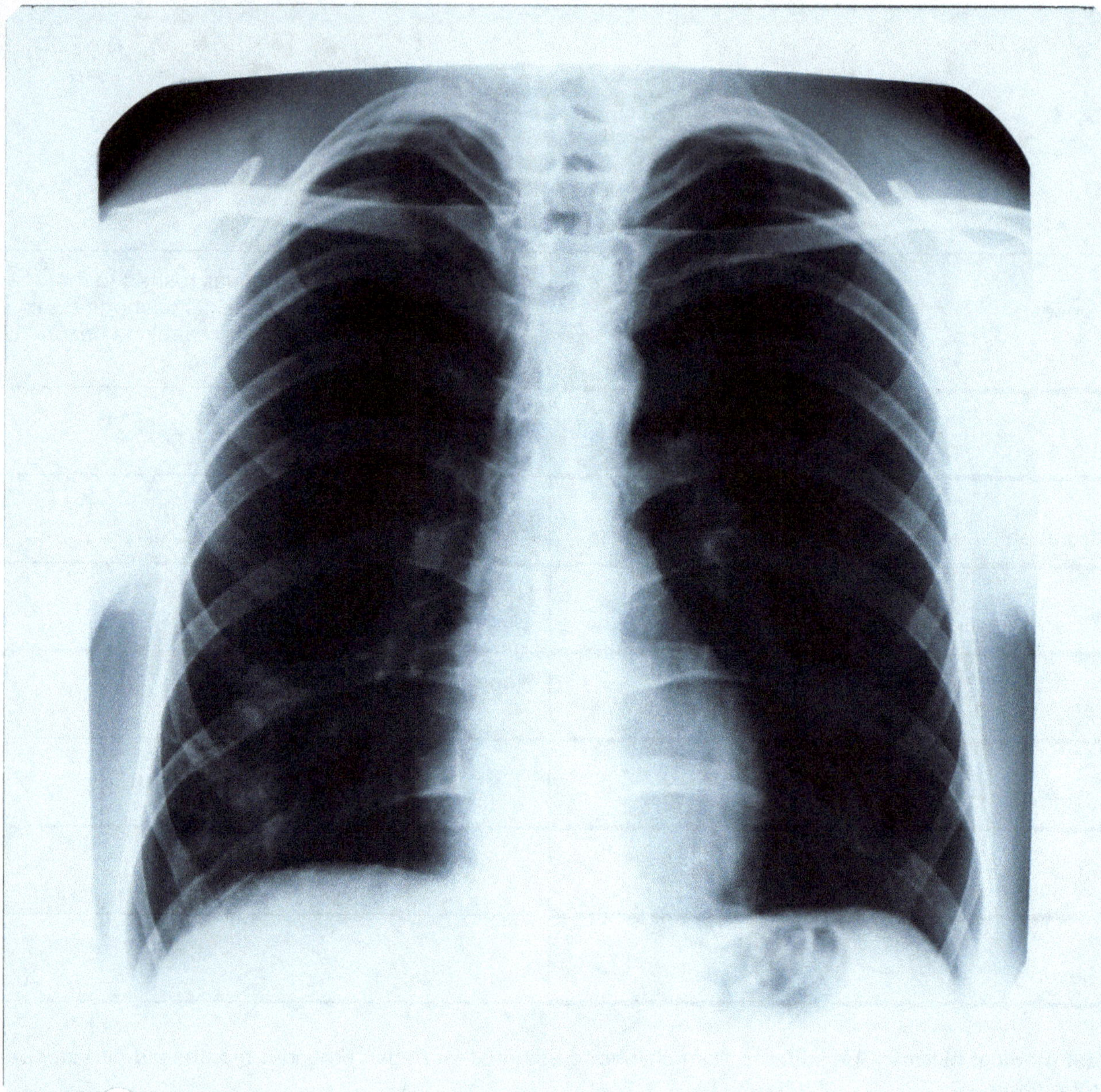

Figure 8.1 Hyperinflated Lung X-ray

Chest X-ray displays hyperinflation. This is most often seen in patients with chronic obstructive pulmonary disease (COPD) but is also possible with asthmatic patients.

Figure 8.2 Normal Chest X-ray

Arterial Blood Gas (ABG) Test: to identify hypoxemia due to hypoventilation: In the event of an asthma attack, the patient's ABG test results are expected to coincide with the acidosis indicated in the abnormal ABG column of the chart that follows:

Value	Normal	Abnormal	
pH	7.35–7.45	<7.35 (acidosis)	>7.45 (alkalosis)
PaO2	>90 mm Hg	75–89 mm Hg (mild hypoxia)	<75 mm Hg (severe hypoxia)
PaCO2	35–45 mm Hg	<35 mm Hg (alkalosis)	>45 mm Hg (acidosis)
HCO3-	18–24 mEq/L	<18 mEq/L (acidosis)	>24 mEq/L (alkalosis)

Auscultation: for breath sounds

Step 3: Based on the collective information from the patient's presentation, diagnostic tests, and medical history, what is your decision regarding treating the patient? Why?

Acute asthma attack induced by ibuprofen. Bronchodilators are appropriate treatment for alleviating the symptoms.

1. Intravenous magnesium and albuterol sulfate inhalers
2. Avoidance of aspirin containing drugs
3. A corticosteroid inhaler to strengthen and maintain respiratory function

Step 4: What are the risk factors for having asthma?

1. Genetic factor
2. Family history
3. Allergens

Step 5: What have you learned from this case?

Image Credits

Fig. 8.1: Copyright © 2014 Depositphotos/deymosd.

Fig. 8.2: Frank Galliard, https://radiopaedia.org/cases/normal-chest-x-ray?lang=us. Copyright © 2010 by Radiopaedia.org.

Chapter 9

Cardiovascular System: Case 1

Onset	A 57-year-old Cuban male feels malaise for 3 months but no pain.
Location	Whole body
Duration	3 months
Characteristic	None
Alleviating Factors	
Aggravating Factors	
Timing	
Severity	

The patient's height is 5′8″. He has a history of diabetes and kidney stones. He has had high cholesterol for 2 years.

Family history: diabetes, cardiovascular diseases, hypertension, and kidney dysfunctions

The patient signed up for a free 3D angiogram in December 2022. In June 2023, the patient had a 3D angiogram and cardiac catheterization. In July 2023, an appointment was made with his surgeon. The surgery was scheduled on August 7, 2023.

Coronary arteries provide blood supply to the heart.

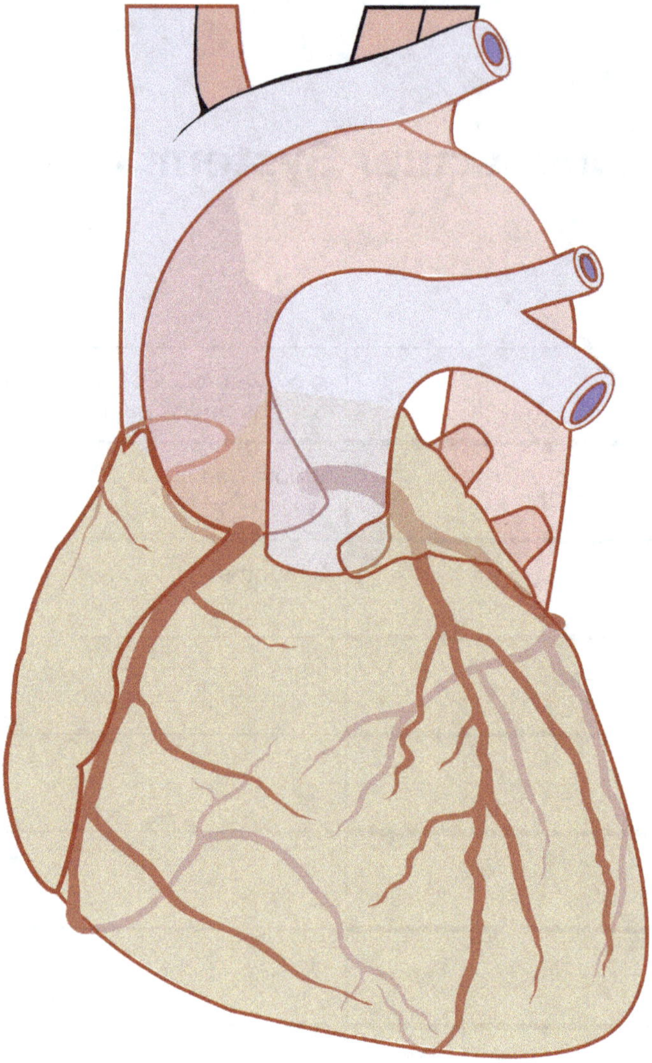

Figure 9.1 Coronary Arteries

Step 1: What are possible diagnoses (3–5)?

1. Coronary artery disease
2. Myocardial infarction
3. Diabetes

Step 2: Based on the medical history, what diagnostic tests should you order?

3D Rotational Angiography is a reliable technique to reconstruct the multidirectional representation of coronary arteries. Atherosclerosis is a blockage of plaque consisting of lipids, calcium, and possible clots. The formation of atherosclerosis is related to factors including diet, exercise, and stress.

Findings:

- Right coronary artery (RCA) is 100% blocked.
- Posterior descending artery (PDA) is 100% blocked.
- Acute marginal artery is 90% blocked.

- Left anterior descending artery is 80% blocked.

Step 3: Based on the collective information from the patient presentation, diagnostic tests, and medical history, what is your decision regarding treating the patient? Why?

A double coronary artery bypass grafting (CABG) surgery is needed based on the evaluation.

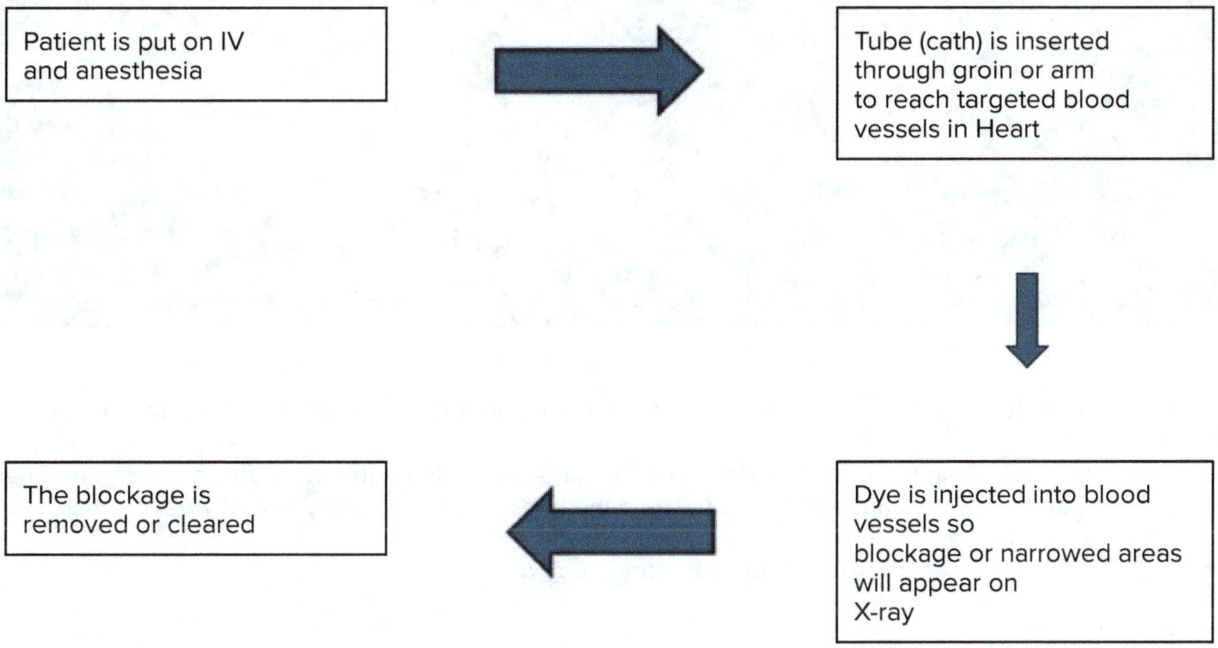

Figure 9.2 *Cardiac Catheterization*

The CABG procedure includes the following steps:

1. Intubation and ventilation support
2. Intravenous lines
3. Urinary catheter
4. Sternotomy
5. Exposure of the heart
6. Temporary inhibition of the heart
7. Placement on a cardiopulmonary bypass machine
8. Harvest of blood vessels.
9. Restarting of the heart and powering off of bypass machine
10. Closure of incisions

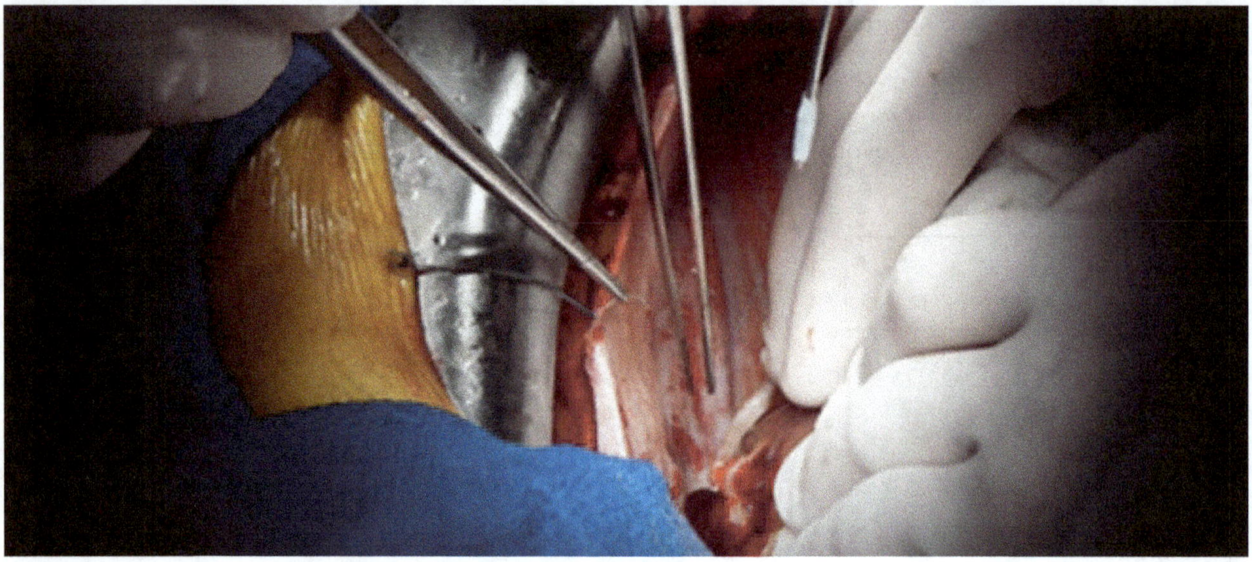

Figure 9.3 Cardiac Catheterization

A cardiac catheterization was performed, but a stent could not be placed due to too much plaque in the arteries.

The patient stayed in the hospital for 5 days. He started to walk the morning after the surgery. Chest tubes were taken out 3 days after the surgery. The patient made a full recovery after 8 weeks. Small meals were provided and eaten.

Step 4: What are the risk factors for having coronary artery disease?

1. Family history
2. Hypertension
3. Diabetes
4. Sedentary lifestyle
5. High-salt, high-lipid foods

Step 5: What have you learned from this case?

Prevention tips:

1. Do not smoke.
2. Eat healthy foods!
3. Weight management
4. Exercise
5. Stress management

Image Credits

Fig. 9.1: Copyright © 2010 by Patrick J. Lynch and Mikael Häggström, M.D. (CC BY-SA 3.0) at https://commons.wikimedia.org/wiki/File:Coronary_arteries.svg.

Chapter 10

Endocrine System: Case 2

Onset	A 50-year-old African American woman has type 2 diabetes, which was diagnosed in 2003.
Location	
Duration	20 years
Characteristic	None
Alleviating Factors	
Aggravating Factors	
Timing	
Severity	

Type 2 diabetes was diagnosed in 2003 after months of experiencing numbness, tingling, and extreme thirst. A treatment plan began in 2013 that included taking metformin, monitoring body weight, exercising, and limiting carbohydrate intake. In 2018, the patient started insulin treatment, discontinued metformin treatment, and continued with low carbohydrate intake as well as exercise.

HbA1c and Glucose measurements:

- 01/2007: 5.8 (HbA1c)
- 03/2016: 8.4 (HbA1c)
- 09/2016: 9 (HbA1c); 256 mg/dL (glucose)
- 10/2016: 200–250 mg/dL (glucose)
- 02/2017: 7 (HbA1c)
- 03/2017: 7.5 (HbA1c)

- 08/2017: 7.5 (HbA1c)
- 11/2017: 6.8 (HbA1c); 80–174 mg/dL with an average of 130 mg/dL (after meal) (glucose)
- 01/2018: 7.5 (HbA1c)
- 10/2018: 7.9 (HbA1c)
- 2019: 7.9 (HbA1c)
- 1/2020: 8.2 (HbA1c)
- 11/2020: 7.7 (HbA1c)
- 04/2021: 8.3 (HbA1c)
- 7/2021: 8.4 (HbA1c); 180 mg/dL (fasting glucose)
- 02/2022: 8.4 (HbA1c); multiple episodes of hypoglycemia (average glucose level is 88 mg/dL)
- 03/2022: hypoglycemia
- 06/2022: 6.1 (HbA1c)
- 01/2023: 6.2 (HbA1c)
- 05/2023: 4–5.6 (HbA1c)
- 09/2023: 5.8 (HbA1c)
- 10/2023: mild hyperglycemia

Other conditions:

- 09/03/2016: Vitamin D deficiency
- 01/2017: Hypercalcemia
- 03/2017: Cholesterol of 148 mg/dL (normal range: 100–200 mg/dL); Triglycerides of 166 mg/dL (normal range: 0–199 mg/dL); LDL of 82 mg/ dL (normal range: 65–160 mg/dL); HDL of 33 mg/dL (normal is > or = to 40 mg/dL)
- 08/2017: Back pain
- 6/10/2018: Hyperglycemia and ketonuria
- 10/2018: Slight hypertension
- 12/2018: Menopause
- 1/2020: Chest pain when walking for more than 3 miles
- 06/2021: Albumin/creatinine ratio was 7.4
- 11/2021: Vitamin D deficiency
- 03/2022: Occasional tingling in hands and feet
- 06/26/2022: Retinopathy (both myopia and presbyopia)
- 06/2023: Lost 60 lb in the past month

Microalbuminuria is the earliest clinically detectable sign of diabetic nephropathy. The urinary albumin is between 30 and 300 mg/d, or the albumin/creatinine ratio is between 2 and 20 mg/mmol.

Step 1: Based on the information from the patient presentation, diagnostic tests, and medical history, what is your decision regarding treating the patient? Why?

Diet: The patient is recommended to eat fewer calories and carbohydrates to reduce body weight. At the same time, snacks are necessary to maintain a normal glucose level.

Daily exercise is also recommended to reduce body weight.

Foot Ulcer

We have an Asian male patient, who is 74 years old and has a type 2 diabetes history of 29 years. A foot ulcer was noticed on the index toe of the left foot around the distal interphalangeal joint. The ulcer had been there for about 3 weeks without an obvious improvement. No bleeding and no pain or other abnormal senses.

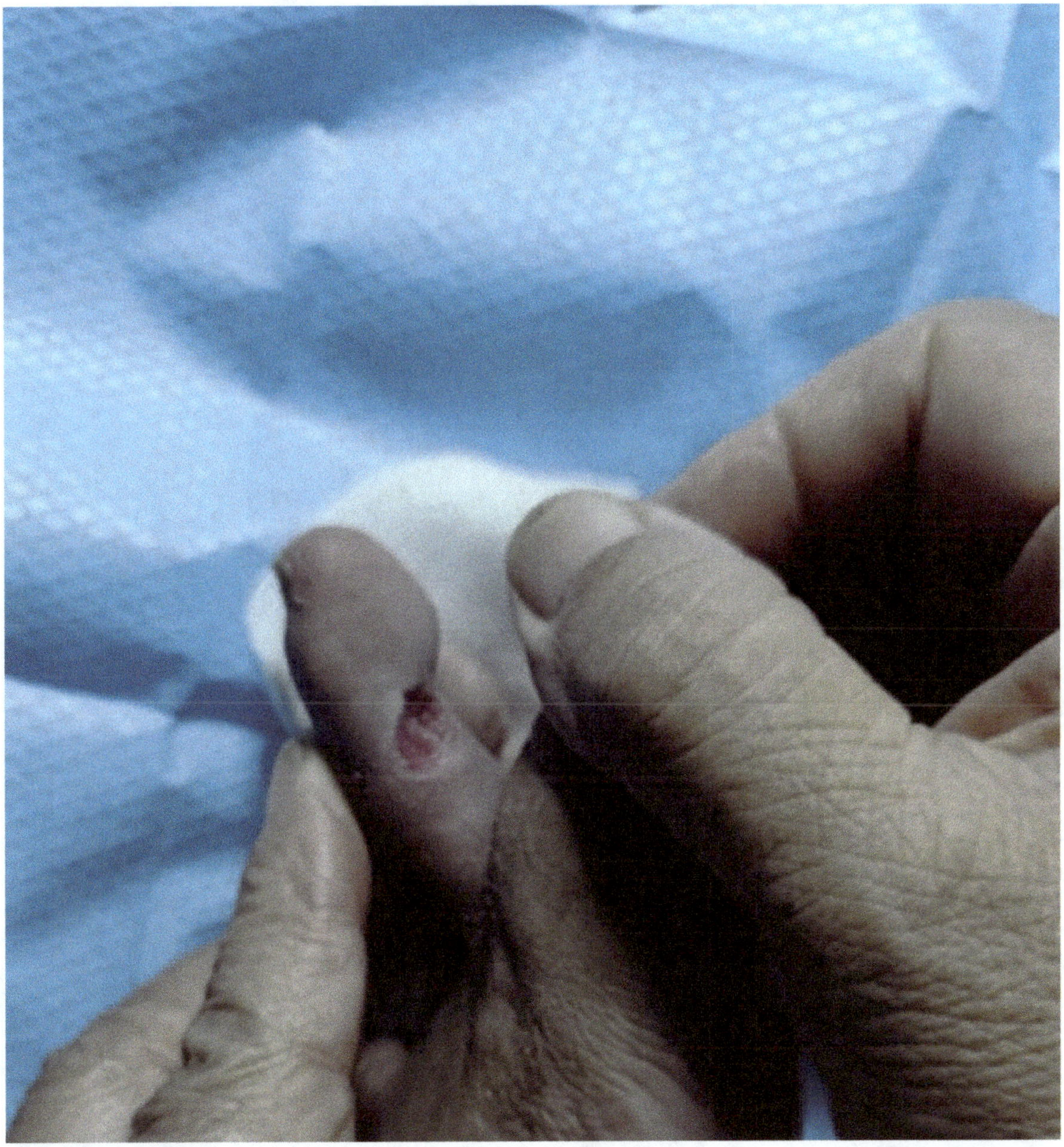

Figure 10.1 Foot Ulcer

An X-ray was taken to rule out osteomyelitis.

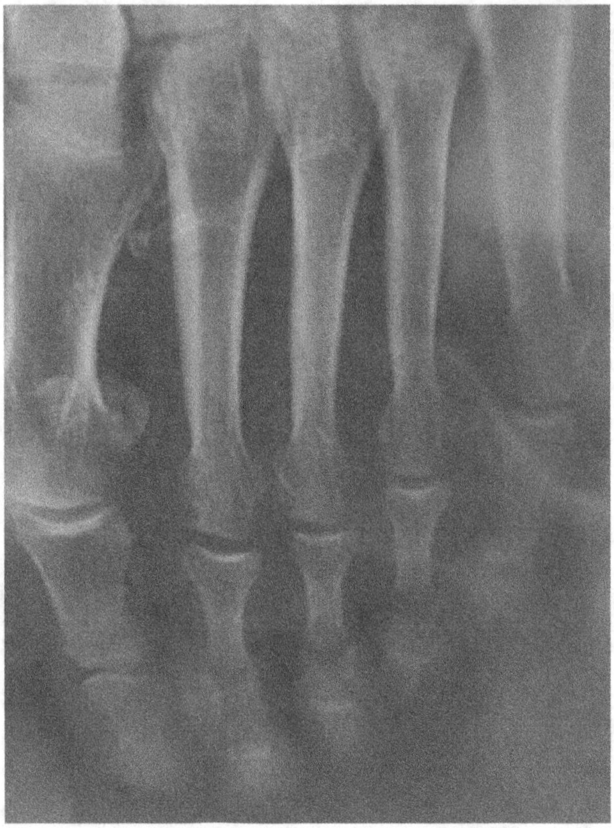

Figure 10.2 Foot X-ray

Image Credits

Fig. 13.2: Mikael Häggström, M.D., https://commons.wikimedia.org/wiki/File:Tissue_selection_from_skin_excision_with_lesion_less_than_4_mm_with_benign_appearance.png, 2019.

Fig. 13.4a: Copyright © 2005 by Kauczuk (CC BY-SA 3.0) at https://commons.wikimedia.org/wiki/File:Squamous_cells.jpg.

Chapter 11

Cardiovascular System: Case 2

Onset	A 22-year-old White female complains of palpation, dizziness/fainting, and chest pain for about 4–6 weeks.
Location	Chest
Duration	4–6 weeks
Characteristic	Occasional, irregular
Alleviating Factors	Pleural involvement
Aggravating Factors	Deep breathing
Timing	Intermittent
Severity	Low-moderate (little interference with daily activities

PLEASE INDICATE WHETHER OR NOT YOU HAVE HAD ANY OF THE FOLLOWING CONDITIONS:

INDICATE:	YES	NO	INDICATE:	YES	NO
Chest Pain / Angina	✓		Gout		✓
Coronary Artery Disease		✓	Dizziness / Fainting	✓	
Heart Murmur		✓	Epilepsy		✓
Heart Attack		✓	Anxiety		✓
Bypass Surgery		✓	Glaucoma / Eye Disorders		✓
Angioplasty (Balloon)		✓	Thyroid Disease or Problem		✓
Heart Rhythm Disturbance	✓		Shortness of Breath		✓
Stent		✓	Asthma		✓
Heart Valve Surgery		✓	COPD / Emphysema		✓
Carotid Blockage		✓	Peptic Ulcer		✓
Leg Circulation Problems		✓	Pancreatitis		✓
Stroke / TIA		✓	Gallbladder Disease		✓
Congenital Heart Disease		✓	Liver Disease, Jaundice, Hepatitis		✓
Rheumatic Heart Disease		✓	Intestinal Problems (Colitis), Etc.		✓
Congestive Heart Failure		✓	Kidney Disease		✓
Heart Palpitations	✓		Urinary Problems		✓
Leg Pain While Walking		✓	Fatigue		✓
Aneurysm		✓	Anemia		✓
Pacemaker or Defibrillator		✓	Bleeding Disorder		✓
High Cholesterol		✓	Arthritis		✓
High Triglycerides		✓	Cancer		✓
High Blood Pressure		✓	HIV/ AIDS		✓
Diabetes		✓	Psychiatric Problems		✓
Abdominal Pain / Fullness		✓	Fever / Chills / Sweats		✓
Mitral Valve Prolapse		✓	Lower Extremity Swelling		✓

Figure 11.1 A table titled "Please Indicate Whether or Not You Have Had Any of the Following Condition" that lists medical conditions along with a column for "Yes" and a column for "No". Chest pain/angina, heart rhythm disturbance, heart palpitations, and dizziness/fainting are marked with a checkmark in the "Yes" column while the rest of the conditions are marked with a checkmark in the "No" column.

Family history: All grandparents have high blood pressure and high cholesterol. Circulation problems in low extremities were seen in one grandmother. One grandfather had a stroke in his 80s. Heart attack and heart bypass occurred with one grandfather in his 50s. Pacemaker was installed in one grandfather in his 70s.

PROBLEM	FAMILY MEMBER / MEMBERS
Stroke	Grandfather 80's
Heart Attack	Grandfather 50's
Heart Bypass	Grandfather 50s
Angioplasty / Stent	Grandfather
Diabetes	
High Blood Pressure	all grandparents
Cholesterol / Triglycerides	all grandparents
Leg Circulation Problems	Grandmother
Carotid (Neck) Blockage	
Pacemaker	Grandfather 70's

Figure 11.2 Family Medical History

Paroxysmal supraventricular tachycardia (PSVT) is an intermittent arrhythmia of the heart due to irregular electrical signals from above ventricles that cause abnormally rapid contractions of the ventricles. While altering lifestyle can improve PSVT, medical intervention is always necessary.

Step 1: What are possible diagnoses (3–5)?

- PSVT
- Angina
- Myocardial infarction

Step 2: Based on the medical history, what diagnostic tests should you order?

Test Name	In Range	Out Of Range	Reference Range	Lab
COMPREHENSIVE METABOLIC PANEL				AT
GLUCOSE	74		65-99 mg/dL Fasting reference interval	
UREA NITROGEN (BUN)	9		7-20 mg/dL	
CREATININE	0.73		0.50-1.00 mg/dL	
eGFR NON-AFR. AMERICAN	119		> OR = 60 mL/min/1.73m2	
eGFR AFRICAN AMERICAN	138		> OR = 60 mL/min/1.73m2	
BUN/CREATININE RATIO	NOT APPLICABLE		6-22 (calc)	
SODIUM	139		135-146 mmol/L	
POTASSIUM		**3.7 L**	3.8-5.1 mmol/L	
CHLORIDE	104		98-110 mmol/L	
CARBON DIOXIDE	22		20-32 mmol/L	
CALCIUM	9.5		8.9-10.4 mg/dL	
PROTEIN, TOTAL	7.0		6.3-8.2 g/dL	
ALBUMIN	4.5		3.6-5.1 g/dL	
GLOBULIN	2.5		2.0-3.8 g/dL (calc)	
ALBUMIN/GLOBULIN RATIO	1.8		1.0-2.5 (calc)	
BILIRUBIN, TOTAL	0.6		0.2-1.1 mg/dL	
ALKALINE PHOSPHATASE		**43 L**	47-176 U/L	
AST	21		12-32 U/L	
ALT	18		5-32 U/L	
MAGNESIUM	1.8		1.5-2.5 mg/dL	AT
TSH		**4.45 H**	mIU/L Reference Range 1-19 Years 0.50-4.30 Pregnancy Ranges First trimester 0.26-2.66 Second trimester 0.55-2.73 Third trimester 0.43-2.91	AT
T4, FREE	1.1		0.8-1.4 ng/dL	AT
T3, TOTAL	150		86-192 ng/dL	AT
CBC (INCLUDES DIFF/PLT)				AT
WHITE BLOOD CELL COUNT	7.3		3.8-10.8 Thousand/uL	
RED BLOOD CELL COUNT	4.82		3.80-5.10 Million/uL	
HEMOGLOBIN	15.1		11.7-15.5 g/dL	
HEMATOCRIT		**45.2 H**	35.0-45.0 %	
MCV	93.8		80.0-100.0 fL	
MCH	31.3		27.0-33.0 pg	
MCHC	33.4		32.0-36.0 g/dL	
RDW	11.3		11.0-15.0 %	
PLATELET COUNT	249		140-400 Thousand/uL	
MPV	10.7		7.5-12.5 fL	
ABSOLUTE NEUTROPHILS	4709		1500-7800 cells/uL	
ABSOLUTE LYMPHOCYTES	1847		850-3900 cells/uL	
ABSOLUTE MONOCYTES	672		200-950 cells/uL	
ABSOLUTE EOSINOPHILS	51		15-500 cells/uL	
ABSOLUTE BASOPHILS	22		0-200 cells/uL	
NEUTROPHILS	64.5		%	

Figure 11.3 Lab Test Results

Elevated TSH can lead to rapid or irregular heartbeat.
Echocardiogram to rule out structural or mechanical issues

M-Mode		M-Mode	
IVSd	0.8 cm	RVIDd	2.1 am
LVIDb	4.4 cm	Ao Diam	2.9 cm
LVPWd	0.8 cm	LA Diam	2.9 cm
LVIDs	2.7 cm		

Impression

: 2-D, M-Mode, and Color Doppler imaging was performed. This was a technically adequate study. Mitral valve structure is normal. No mitral regurgitation. The tricuspid valve structure is normal. Trace tricuspid regurgitation with RVSP of 20-25 mmHg. The aortic valve structure is normal. No aortic regurgitation. The pulmonic valve structure is normal. There is no pulmonic regurgitation. The left ventricular size is normal. Left ventricular wall size is normal. There is normal global left ventricular function with an ejection fraction >55%. The diastolic function is normal. The right ventricle is normal in size. The right ventricular wall thickness is normal. The right ventricular systolic function is normal. The left atrial size is normal. The right atrial size is normal. There is no pericardial effusion. The aortic root size is normal. Inferior vena cava is normal.

Summary

1. This was a technically adequate study.
2. Trace tricuspid regurgitation with RVSP of 20-25 mmHg.
3. There is normal global left ventricular function with an ejection fraction >55%.
4. The diastolic function is normal.

Figure 11.4 *Echocardiogram Results*

Echocardiography is used to see heart valve movements, blood flow, and cardiac output. Most heart functions were in normal range, with trace tricuspid regurgitation. Tricuspid valve regurgitation causes abnormal heart rhythms.

Event/Loop Monitor Report

- Dates monitored: 05/23/19–06/21/19
- Number of transmissions: 9
- Impression: 1. Sinus rhythm; 2. Sinus tachycardia
- Patient wore an event monitor for 19 days (7 days omitted due to equipment error).
- Patient was tachycardic for 21% of the monitored time. No evidence of atrial fibrillation had been observed.

Summary:

The patient's monitoring period was 05/23/2019-06/21/2019. Baseline sample showed Sinus Tachycardia w/PVCs (12 in 1min) with a heart rate of 123.2 bm. There were 0 critical, 1 serious, and 8 stable events that occurred. The report analysis of the critical, serious, stable and manually triggered events are listed below.

Automatically detected events:

1 Serious: Sinus Rhythm, Ventricular Tachycardia (5 Beats) with/Couplet
PVCs/Bigeminal PVCs/PVCs (9 in 1 min)

1 Stable: Sinus Tachycardia w/PVCs (12 in 1 min)

1 Stable: Sinus Rhythm w/PVCs (8 in 1 min)/Artifact

1 Stable: Sinus Arrythmia w/Artifact/Lead Loss

1 Stable: Sinus Rhythm w/PSVT/PVCs (5 in 1 min)/Artifact

Manually Detected Events:

1 Stable: Sinus Tachycardia, Sinus Arrythmia w/PVCs (4 in 1 min)/Artifact
No Symptoms Received

1 Stable: Sinus Tachycardia w/PVCs (10 in 1 min)/Artifact
None of Accidental Push

1 Stable: Sinus Rhythm w/MF PVCs (6 in a min)/Artifact
None Reported

1 Stable: Sinus Tachycardia w/PVCs (5 in 1 min)/Artifact/Lead Loss
None Reported

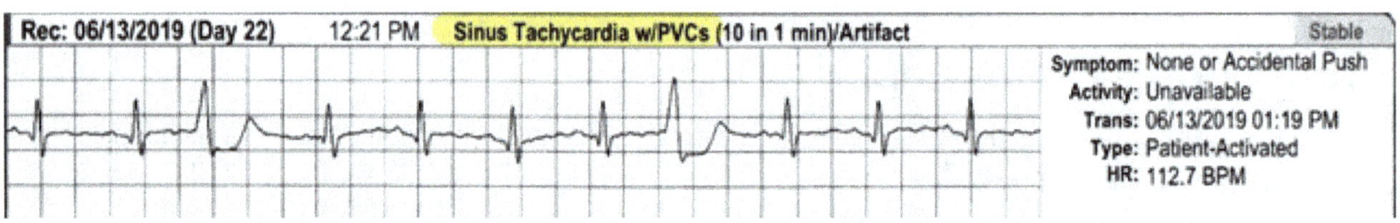

Figure 11.5a Sinus Tachycardia with PVCs

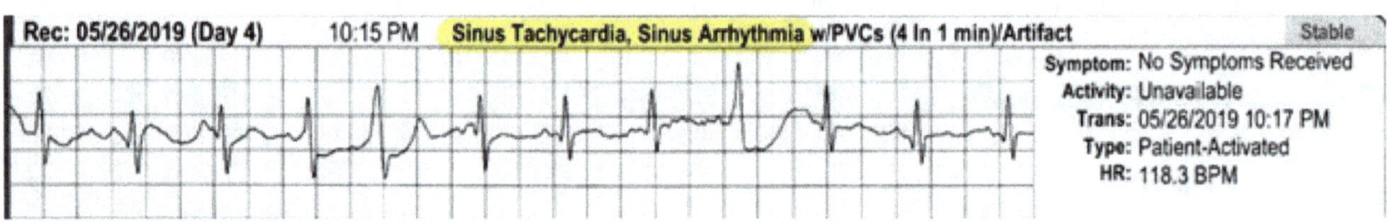

Figure 11.5b Sinus Tachycardia, Sinus Arrhythmia with PVCs

Step 3: Based on the information on the patient presentation, diagnostic tests, medical history, what is your decision to treat the patient? Why?

PSVT can be treated with **beta blockers**.

Acebutolol is more selective for beta-1 receptors over beta-2 receptors. Beta 1 receptors are found in cardiac muscle and have no effects on bronchial or smooth vascular smooth muscle.

Also, acebutolol has partial agonist activity so this leads to less pronounced negative impact on cardiac contractility compared to other beta-blockers. This drug is preferred because of its cardioselectivity. It has a selective effect on heart rate and rhythm.

Another alternative would be a calcium channel blocker. **Verapamil** and **diltiazem** work by inhibiting calcium entry into the cells of the heart, leading to decreased contractility and a slower heart rate. They have a specific effect on the AV node which is involved in the reentrant circuits responsible for SVT. By slowing conduction through the AV node, both medications can help restore a normal heart rhythm.

Alternative treatment/therapies:

1. Valsalva maneuver: pushing air out with your nose and mouth closed. This increases pressure in the eyes and belly.
2. Carotid sinus massage: applying firm pressure on the carotid sinus for 10–15 seconds on both sides of the neck.

What if vagal maneuvers are not working?

Quick relief of SVT involves using adenosine. It is administered intravenously. It works rapidly and has less potential for side effects.

A surgical option is catheter ablation- uses cold or heat energy to create tiny scars in the heart to block faulty electric signals. This restores the normal heart rhythm.

Step 4: What are the risk factors for having PSVT?

- Family history

Hypertension Lifestyle modification recommendations:

- Eat a healthy diet rich in fruits, vegetables, and whole grains.
- Limit salt intake and saturated fat intake.
- Abstain from smoking.
- Manage body weight.
- Avoid or limit alcohol.
- Reduce stress. Participating in yoga, meditation, or relaxation techniques can reduce stress.

Step 5: What have you learned from this case?

The electrical conduction pathway of the heart starts at the sinoatrial node (SA), moves to the atrioventricular (AV) node (at which point the electrical signal is delayed for around 100 milliseconds to allow the atria to contract and empty before ventricular contraction), to the Bundle of His, and then goes from the R/L bundle branches to the Purkinje fibers.

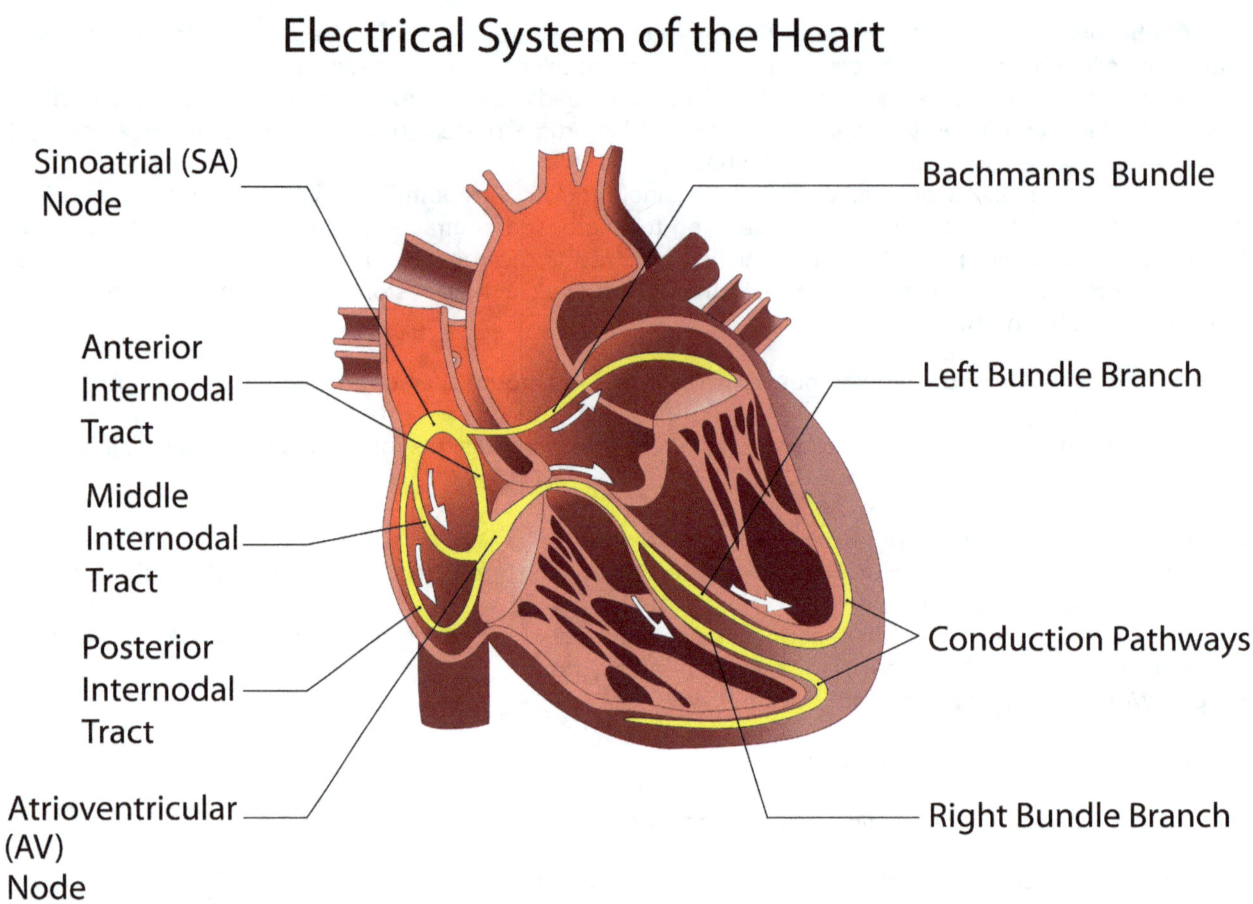

Figure 11.6 Electrical System of the Heart

Supraventricular Tachycardia Pathophysiology

In SVT, the primary electrical signal does not come from the SA node. Instead, it originates from another part of the atria or from the AV node. As a result, an area outside the AV node begins to fire signals very quickly. This causes a rapid heartbeat of around 100 beats per minute, shortening the amount of time the ventricles have to fill with blood. If the heart rate is fast enough, the heart may be unable to pump enough blood to the rest of the body.

Prognosis

The prognosis for paroxysmal SVT cases with no structural heart disease is reasonably good.

SVT is considered a heart arrhythmia, so it may come on suddenly and last anywhere from a few seconds to several days.

Patients may experience anxiety, a sense of doom, and perhaps hemodynamic compromise.

If there are no other factors that interfere with heart function, the risk of sudden death with paroxysmal SVT is extremely small.

Image Credits

Chapter 12

Inflammation (Immune System): Case 1

Onset	The patient is a 19-year-old White female. Strep throat was left untreated in 2017. Yearly strep throat occurred until 2019; then it became a monthly event. Rheumatic fever occurred in the summer of 2019.
Location	Throat, face, joints, arms, and heart
Duration	Rheumatic fever (2019–2020) with intermittent inflammatory episodes
Characteristic	Joints are red, swollen and warm to touch; swollen face and eyes; rash was seen in face and neck; heart palpitations; fever
Alleviating Factors	
Aggravating Factors	Deep breathing
Timing	Strep throat/chronic tonsilitis (2017–2020)
Severity	Moderate to severe

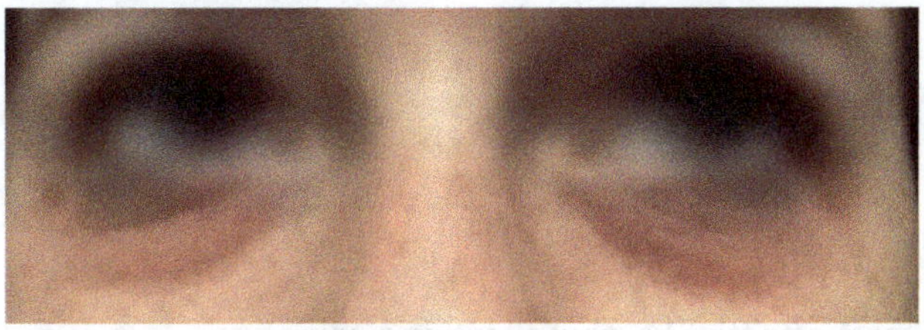

Figure 12.1 Rashes (under the Eyes)

Step 1: What are possible diagnoses (3–5)?

- Rheumatic fever
- Tonsillitis
- COVID-19

Step 2: Based on the medical history, what diagnostic tests should you order?

A dermatologist checked the skin rash, which was diagnosed as idiopathic.

Blood tests: antibody titer test; acute phase reactants; erythrocyte sedimentation rate; C-reactive protein

Diagnostic Tests:

- Throat culture: multiple (monthly) strep A+ throat cultures were performed between 2019 and 2020 by the primary physician.
- Antibody titer test: anti-streptolysin O titer = 325 IU/ml
- Blood culture: acute phase reactants, erythrocyte sedimentation rate, a higher C-reactive protein level than normal range
- Stress test: tachycardia and palpitations were observed with exertion.

Step 3: Based on the information on the patient presentation, diagnostic tests, medical history, what is your decision to treat the patient? Why?

Antibiotics/Penicillin Shot: a 3-day Z-pack (azithromycin) and a round of clarithromycin were given to treat the strep A pharyngitis. The treatment was unsuccessful due to the drug resistance of the infection. Next, a penicillin shot was administered for the strep, which was successful, but too late to prevent the onset of RF.

Side Effects: pain, tenderness, and hematoma at the injection site of the penicillin shot; stomach upset and antibiotic resistance were seen with the use of the amoxicillin; severe headaches, throat pain, fever, and loss of appetite were seen after the tonsillectomy; nausea, difficulty sleeping, and disorientation were associated with the use of oxycodone/hydrocodone.

Pain Killers and Anti-inflammatory Medications: NSAIDs; rest, ice, compress, and elevate (RICE) for joints; a cold compress on inflamed eyes; gentle cleansers and aloe vera on the face to relieve itching and heat

Tonsillectomy: Once it was clear that the tonsils were severely infected, the only treatment left was to remove them to prevent recurrence. Post-operational pain was relieved via opioids (oxycodone, hydrocodone) and oral lidocaine

Step 4: What are the risk factors for contracting rheumatic fever?

1. Recurrent strep throat
2. Female gender

Step 5: What have you learned from this case?

Rheumatic Fever

- An acute systemic inflammatory disease that can result from untreated Streptococcus A infections.
- Rheumatic fever (RF) symptoms commonly include inflamed, painful joints, rashes on the face and neck, and inflammation of heart vessels.

If RF is left untreated, long-term effects and complications can arise:

1. When RF is not treated immediately, rheumatic heart disease can develop. This can weaken and

inflame the heart valves, leading to permanent scarring of the heart and obstructing blood flow. Heart valve damages can appear years after initial infection, which includes but not limited to valve stenosis, ruptured heart valves, atrial fibrillation, and endocarditis.
2. Joint pain due to arthritis arising from RF. The manifestations are swollen, tender, and red joints.
3. Sydenham chorea: Jerky or uncontrollable body movements that can be seen in the hands, feet, and face. Outbursts of unusual behavior and inappropriate laughing or crying can be observed as well.

Strep Throat

- (As known as pharyngitis) A secondary bacterial infection caused by group A beta-hemolytic Streptococcus Pneumoniae invading inflamed mucous membranes.
- Symptoms include fever, swollen throat, headache, and swollen, white-coated tonsils.

In the patient, heart palpitations, tachycardia, and shortness of breath still occur during exercise and sedentary activities. She has commonly observed a HR of 198 bpm on a run of 2–3 minutes or a HR of 120–140 bpm while rest. The probability of recurrence is very low due to the tonsillectomy, which significantly decreases the chances of strep throat infections and RF.

Chapter 13

Integumentary System: Case 1

Onset	The patient is a 53-year-old female. She found a nodule on the inside of the right cheek approximately 3 months ago.
Location	Buccal mucosa
Duration	The nodule is estimated to be in the mouth for at least one year.
Characteristic	Unifocal and hard; 3 cm wide and 13 mm depth
Alleviating Factors	Night guard, eating slowly
Aggravating Factors	Consistent biting, speech, mastication, and teeth brushing
Timing	A diagnosis of squamous cell carcinoma was made on 3/23/2023. Remission was by July 2023.
Severity	Severe

Social history: Former smoker for 19 years; vegetarian

Medical history: No prior history of diabetes

The patient remembered her dental hygienist asking about the cheek, as they thought the patient was biting her cheek and the patient was dismissed without further check.

Step 1: What are possible diagnoses (3–5)?

1. Sore
2. Injuries
3. Cancer

Step 2: Based on the medical history, what diagnostic tests should you order?

Component	Patient Value	Standard Range
Alkaline phosphatase	108 IU/L	35–104 IU/L
ALT w/ P5P	73 IU/L	0–35 IU/L
AST w/ P5P	68 IU/L	0–35 IU/L
Red Blood Cell	5.44 x 10*6/uL	4.20–5.40 x 10*6/uL
Glucose (Point of Care)	183 mg/dL	70–99 mg/dL
HCO3	19 mmol/L	21–29 mmol/L
Calcium Level Total	8.5 mg/dL	8.6–10.4 mg/dL
Albumin Level	3.2 g/dL	3.5–5.0 g/dL

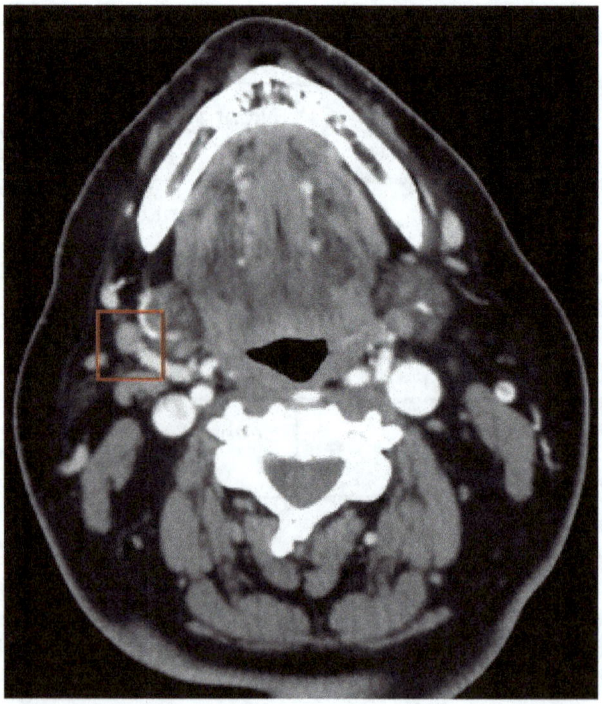

Figure 13.1 Neck CT With Contrast

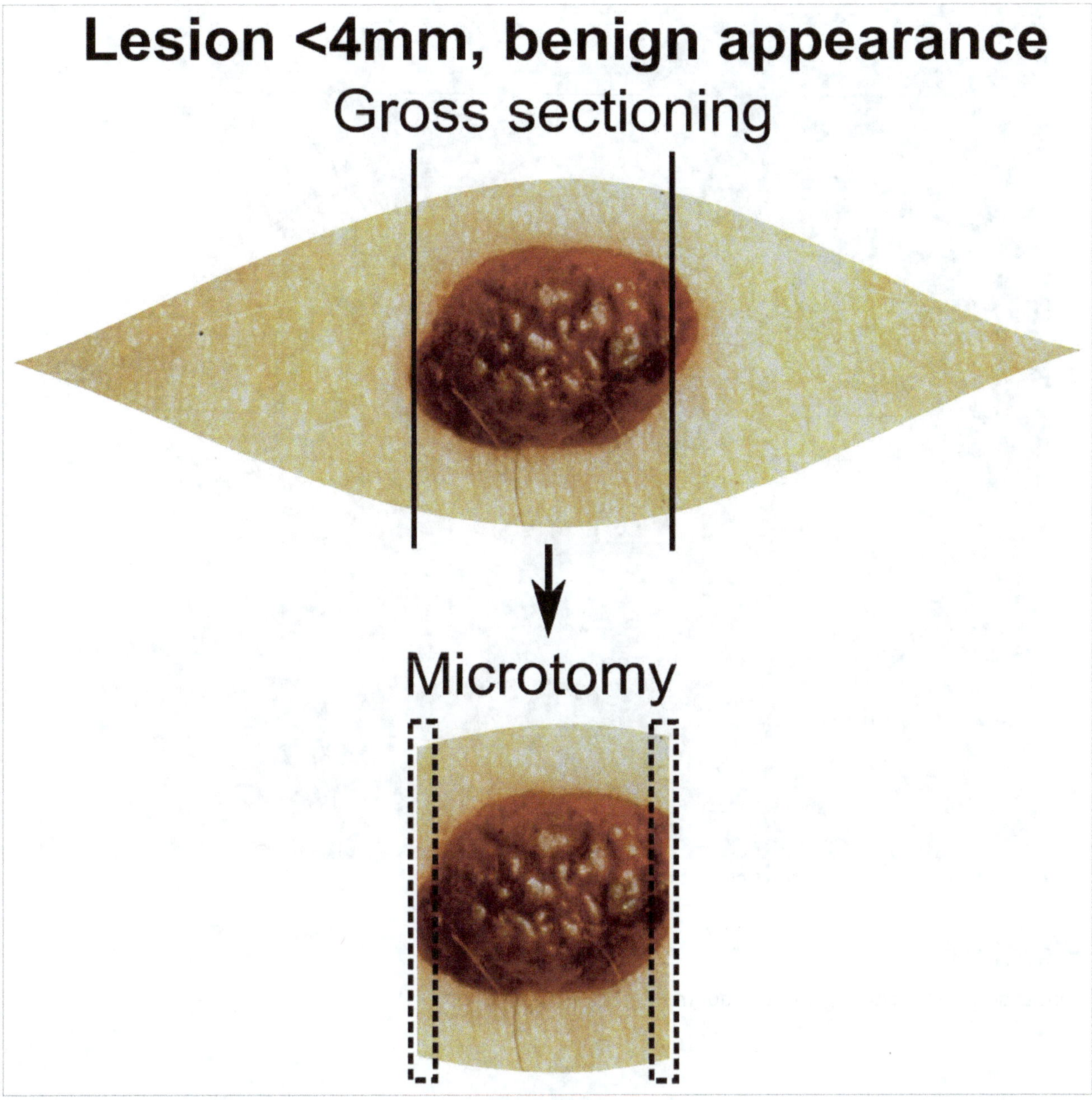

Figure 13.2 Excisional Biopsy

Diagnosis: Stage IV squamous cell carcinoma

The cancer had metastasized to lymph nodes and parotid salivary gland. The severity is related to the delay of the care. Due to the location of the cancer, it was hard to diagnose and caused much pain to the patient.

Step 3: Based on the information on the patient presentation, diagnostic tests, medical history, what is your decision regarding treating the patient? Why?

Surgery: right buccal mucosal resection; skin graft taken from shoulder and arm

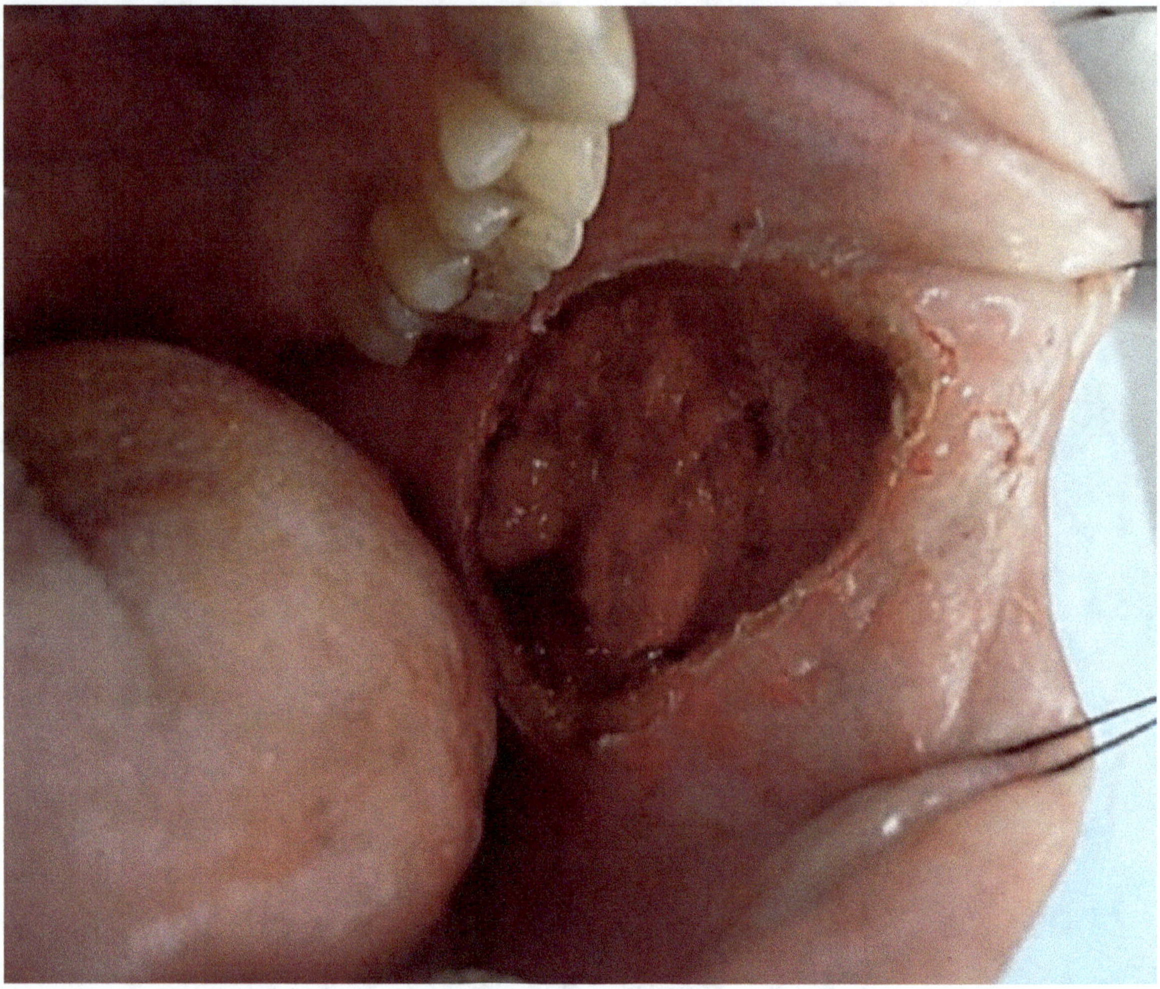

Figure 13.3 Buccal Squamous Cell Carcinoma

Histology

Normal squamous cells (a) versus squamous cell carcinoma (b)

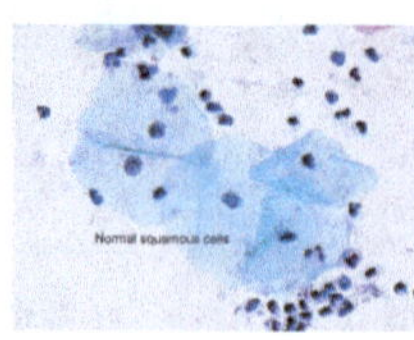

Figure 13.4a Normal Squamous Cells

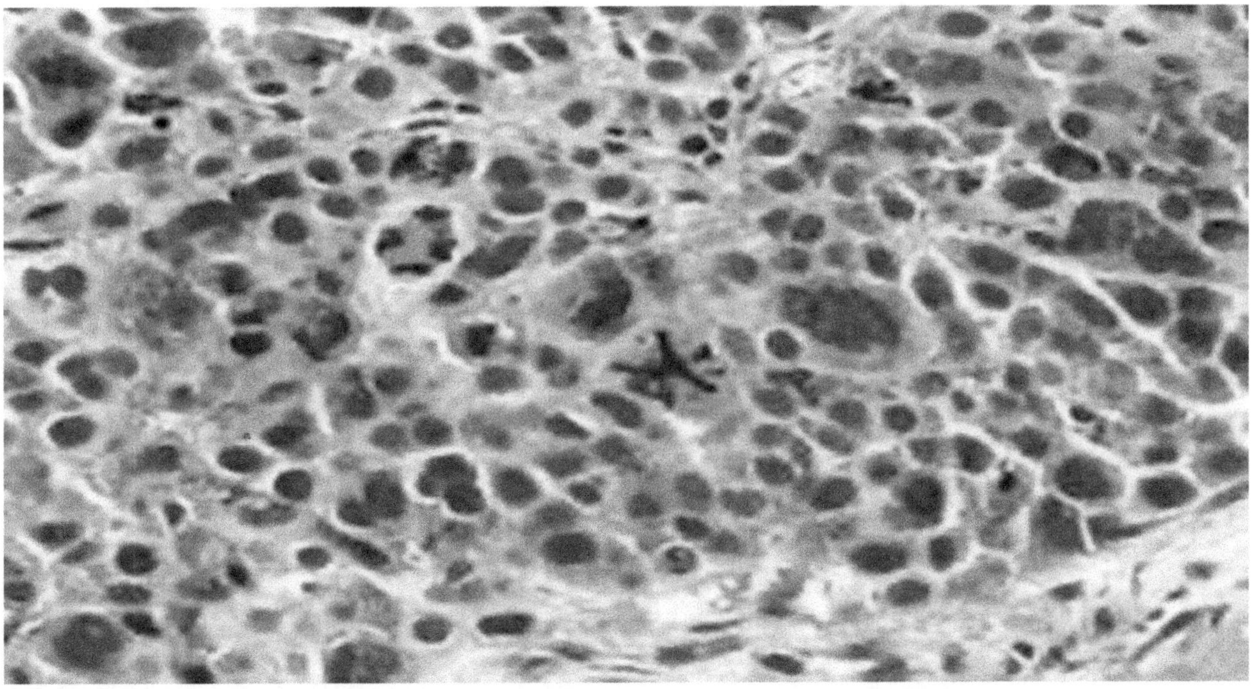

Figure 13.4b Squamous Cell Carcinoma

Post Surgery Therapy: Chemotherapy and radiotherapy for 4 months; nasogastric tube for protein shakes and other nutritional supplements; remission checkup

Medications:

- Amlodipine-benazepril 10 mg: one capsule a day
- Dexamethasone 4 mg: twice a day with meals for 2 days after chemotherapy
- Fluconazole (for thrush): 100 mg; two tablets the day after chemotherapy: one a day on days 2, 3, and 4
- Olanzapine 10 mg: before chemotherapy on day 1 and then as needed after
- Prochlorperazine 10 mg: one tablet every 6 hours as needed
- Acetaminophen 30 mL: every 6 hours through nasogastric tube
- Amlodipine 5 mg: one tablet by feeding tube daily
- Aspirin 81 mg: four tablets daily by feeding tube

Step 4: What are the risk factors for having squamous cell carcinoma?

1. Smoking history
2. Dental hygiene

Step 5: What have you learned from this case?

- Amlodipine-benazepril: Antihypertensive Drug (treat high blood pressure)
    - Common brand: Lotrel
- Dexamethasone: Steroid (treat inflammation)

    - Common brand: Decadron
- Fluconazole: Antifungal (prescribed for treatment of thrush)
    - Common brand: Diflucan
    - Thrush is fungal infection of your mouth from overgrowth of Candida yeast. It is caused by certain medications and antibiotics.
- Olanzapine: Antipsychotic (treat nausea and vomiting from chemotherapy)
    - Common brand: Zyprexa
- Prochlorperazine: Antipsychotic and Antiemetic (treat nausea and vomiting)
    - Common brand: Compazine
- Acetaminophen: Analgesic (treat minor aches and pains, and reduces fever)
    - Common brand: Tylenol
- Amlodipine: Calcium channel blocker (suppress proliferation of cancer cells)
    - Common brand: Norvasc
- Aspirin: Nonsteroidal anti-inflammatory drug and blood thinner (treats pain, fever, headache, and inflammation; prevents spread of cancer)
    - Common brand: Bayer

Prevention

Routine dental care is highly important.

Chapter 14

Nervous System: Case 2

Onset	The patient is a 10-year-old boy. He presented to the ER with a severe laceration above the right eye after being hit in the head with a baseball bat during a ballgame.
Location	Right orbital muscle laceration, lesions of the right temporal and frontal lobe of the brain
Duration	
Characteristic	Headaches, nocturnal seizures
Alleviating Factors	Rest, hydration
Aggravating Factors	Stress, dehydration
Timing	
Severity	Severe

Timeline of Medical History

April 17, 2013: Surgical repair for a 10-year-old boy with a laceration above his right eye after being hit by a baseball bat. An incidental finding was seen on the CT scan and the patient was referred to a neurosurgeon at the Children's of Alabama.

May 2013: an MRI was ordered, and a complete neurological exam was performed. The patient is asymptomatic, and no medication was prescribed.

July 19, 2015: The patient had the first nocturnal seizure. The patient was transported by ambulance to the Children's of Alabama. A CT scan was done.

September 2015: The patient was brought to the Children's of Alabama.by his parents after having a nocturnal seizure. Loading dose of Keppra was given by IV. The patient was sent home with prescribed Keppra.

From October 2015 to May 2016: The dosage of Keppra was increased with each breakthrough nocturnal seizure until a maximum dose of 2,000 mg bid was reached.

From 2016 to January 2017: Trileptal was added. The dosage was increased with each breakthrough seizure until a dose of 650 mg bid was reached.

From 2017 to 2022: The patient was stable on medications. In total, there were four breakthrough seizures.

Side effects related to the medications included the following:

- Frequent headaches diagnosed as migraines in nature
- Issues with venous return in lower extremities that require vein valves to be examined
- Fatigue (from Trileptal?)
- Hair loss
- Weight gain

May 2022: The patient expressed an interest in removing cavernous malformations surgically. The neurosurgeon presented the case to the epilepsy committee at the Children's of Alabama for review and approval.

December 2022: The patient was admitted to the epilepsy monitoring unit at the Children's of Alabama. Grand mal seizure occurred at approximately 11 pm.

February 2023: Annual MRI and neurosurgeon visit. The epilepsy committee approved a dual craniotomy to remove the right frontal and right temporal cavernomas.

November 2023: Presurgical labs completed

December 13, 2023: Dual craniotomy completed at the Children's of Alabama

December 18, 2023: The patient was discharged to home.

What is a cerebral cavernous malformation?

A collection of small, irregularly shaped blood vessels, specifically capillaries, inside the central nervous system. The vessels are enlarged, thinner than normal, less elastic, and can leak. This can be caused by gene mutation or occur with no familial history. Approximately 1 in 100 to 200 people have cavernous malformations (https://www.hopkinsmedicine.org/health/conditions-and-diseases/cavernous-malformations). The most common symptoms include headaches or seizure. The location and number of lesions affect the experiencing of these symptoms.

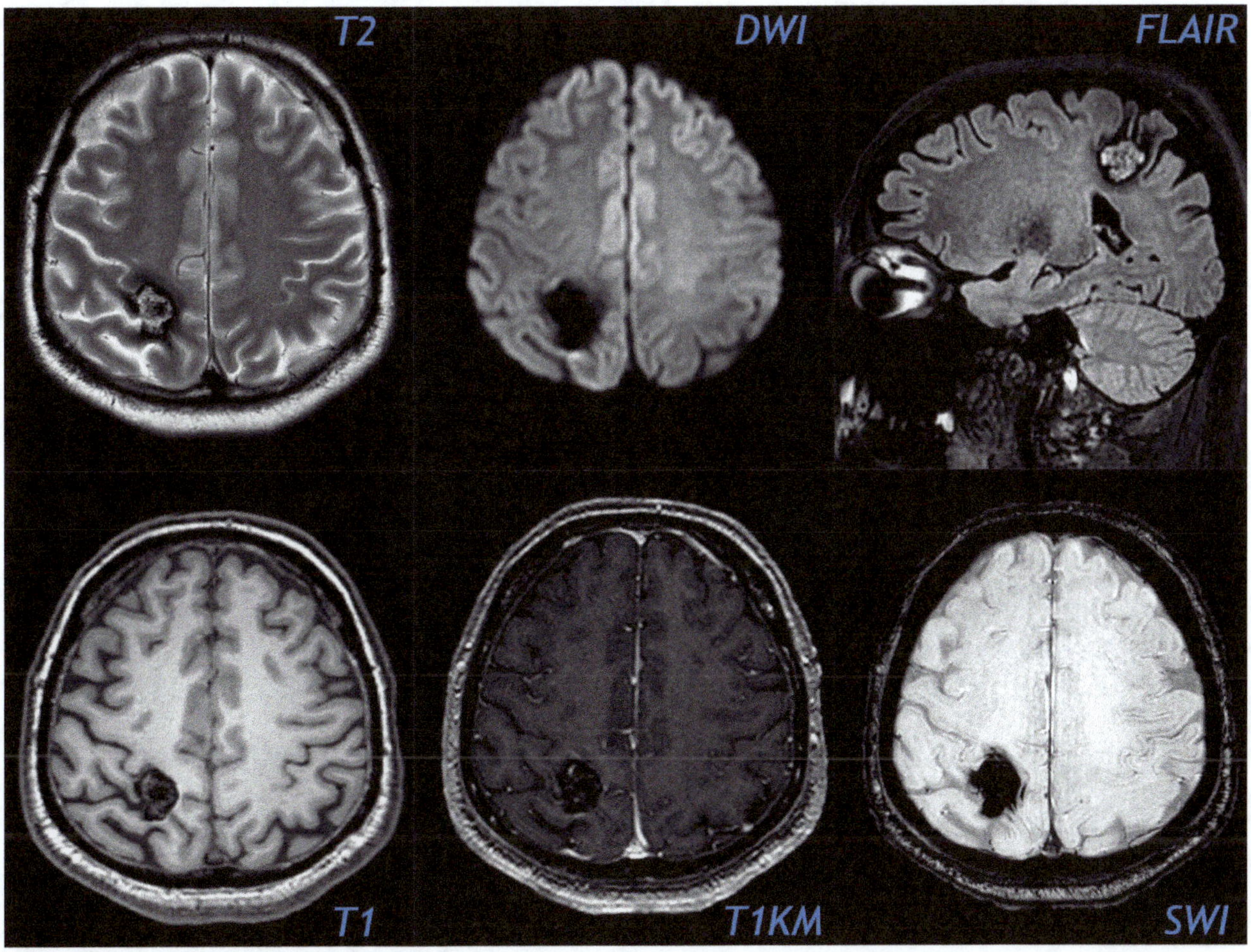

Figure 14.1 Cavernous Malformation

The malformation is not under pressure like arteriovenous malformations. Although there is no risk of aneurysm, they are leaky.

Step 1: What are possible diagnoses (3–5)?

1. Traumatic brain injury
2. Cancer
3. Congenital brain lesion

Step 2: Based on the medical history, what diagnostic tests should you order?

Electroencephalogram (EEG)

MRI (performed every 3 months to monitor the growth in year one (2013–2014), then every 6 months (2015–2016), and later, annually (2017–present). There is no growth/change of the lesions since original findings in 2013. Initial MRI scan indicated that the lesions were located in the right middle frontal gyrus, right superior temporal gyrus, right amygdala, right posterior centrum semiovale, and left superior frontal gyrus. No reduced diffusion within the brain or skull. Normal marrow signal intensity within the skull base, calvarium, and facial skeleton.

Treatment

Nonsurgical treatment started once symptoms started to manifest.

- Nonsurgical treatment with medications: started with Keppra until patient was at maximum dosage without control of nocturnal episodes
- Trileptal added as second medication: symptoms and episodes well controlled with very limited breakthrough episodes
- Epilepsy study done December 2022 to confirm location of lesions: The patient desired to have lesions removed

Presurgical Labs

- Blood Type: O positive
- Activated partial thromboplastin time: 24.5 (normal range 23.5–36.4)
- Prothrombin time: 12.5 (normal range 12.1–14.6)
- CBC with differential: all values within normal ranges
- Fluid balance panel: normal values for all except sodium, which was low at 135 (normal 136–145)

Blood (Venous)Test		Normal Range	Unit
WBC	4.38	3.91–8.77	10*3/uL
RBC	5.45	4.18–5.48	10*6/uL
Hemoglobin	16.7	11.9–15.4	g/dL
Hematocrit	48.2	36.2–46.3	%
MCV	88.4	80–93.6	fL
MCH	30.6	26.5–31.4	pg
MCHC	34.6	31.9–34.8	g/dL
RDWCV	12.2	12.3–14.3	%
RDWSD	39.5	37.8–46.1	fL
Platelet Count	216	140–440	10*3/uL
MPV	8.7	9.7–11.9	fL
nRBC	0	0–0	/100 WBC
Neut	58.7	40.3–74.8	%
Lymph	30.1	12.2–47.1	%
Mono	8.2	4.4–12.3	%
Eos	1.8	0–4.4	%
Baso	0.7	0.0–0.7	%
IG	0.0	0.6	%
AbsNeut	2.57	1.82–7.42	10*3/uL
AbsLymph	1.32	0.85–3	10*3/uL
AbsMono	0.36	0.19–0.77	10*3/uL
AbsEos	0.08	0.03–0.44	10*3/uL
AbsBaso	0.03	0.01–0.05	10*3/uL

Blood (Venous)Test		Normal Range	Unit
AbsIG	0.02	0–0.09	10*3/uL

Surgical intervention was planned for May 2023, but the patient made the decision to postpone after discussion of potential side effects including loss of memory and potential of stroke.

- Dual craniotomy scheduled for December 13, 2023: removal of right temporal and right frontal lobe lesions and surrounding brain tissue
- Post-surgical MRI showed clear margins and removal of lesions

Operative notes for surgery at Children's Hospital of Alabama on December 13, 2023

- Right frontal craniotomy for resection of frontal cavernous malformation
- Right temporal craniotomy for resection of temporal cavernous malformation
- Use of operative microscope for microdissection
- Use of Stealth Neuronavigation
- 20-year-old man who I have been following for some time with multiple intracranial cavernous malformations as well as a spinal cord cavernous malformation. He developed nocturnal epilepsy several years ago and has been managed on seizure medication. Over the past year, he has required multiple seizure medications and has continued to have seizures. In addition, he is having side effects from his seizure medications. He then had long-term EEG monitoring that demonstrated a right frontotemporal onset for his epilepsy, corresponding with his right frontal and right temporal cavernous malformations. His case was reviewed in an epilepsy conference and, given the concordant imaging and EEG data, recommended the option of craniotomy for resection of both right frontal and temporal cavernous malformations to potentially decrease his dependence on AEDs for seizure control. We had a long discussion with his mother regarding this option, and the parents asked that we proceed. We discussed the risks, benefits alternatives of the surgery at length with them, with emphasis on bleeding, infection, CSF leak, need for repeat surgery, stroke, seizures, paralysis, speech deficit, coma and even death. They understood and asked that we proceed.

Description of procedure notable points

- Positioning and preparation to begin surgery took 2 hours
- Surgeon was cognizant of patient outcome and post-surgical stress, choosing the placement for incision that would be best hidden and require the least hair removal
- Use of Marcaine with epinephrine to minimize bleeding from the scalp to help in better visualization of the surgical field
- Bone of the skull was found to be "grayish" in color; sample sent off and no issues identified
- Bur holes drilled to make a 2 x 2 bone flap for access to the dura and brain for frontal resection
- Three additional Bur holes and bone flap made for temporal bone. In addition, had to cut open a small segment of temporalis muscle (Probably the worst post-surgical pain after the headache was the jaw pain.)
- Titanium plates and screws used to put bone flap back in place

Actual Description of the Procedure

After informed consent was obtained, he was brought the operating room and intubated by the anesthesia team. He was carefully positioned supine with his head turned to the left and all bony prominences carefully padded in Mayfield pins. We registered his anatomy with Stealth Neuronavigation with excellent accuracy. We mapped out the entry points for both the right frontal and right temporal lesions. We sketched out an incision, which would go anterior to the ear and then course posteriorly to stay well behind his hairline for the best cosmetic outcome. A small bit of hair was clipped along this, and the scalp was thoroughly prepped with chlorhexidine scrub, alcohol and ChloraPrep prior to sterile draping and placement of bacteriostatic Ioban film. After infiltration of the scalp with 0.25% Marcaine with epinephrine, a 15 blade was used to open the incision extending from just above and anterior to the zygoma in the hairline and then to approximately 2 cm off midline. We first kept the temporalis muscle down and mapped out our opening for our right frontal craniotomy for the right frontal cavernous malformation. A high-speed bur drill was used to make bur holes, and a 2 x 2 cm bone flap was elevated. Of note, the bone was grayish discolored but did not have significant vascularity. The dura was then opened in a cruciate manner. We used the Stealth to locate the appropriate cortical entry site. A small corticectomy was made with bipolar cautery and sharp dissection, and we immediately found ourselves on top of the cavernous malformation. We were able to dissect around this completely and remove it en bloc. There was a small amount of hemosiderin-stained tissue adjacent, which was also removed. We saw no evidence of residual cavernous malformation and no significant hemosiderin-stained tissue with normal-appearing white matter, gray matter, or sulci in all directions. Surgicel was placed over the resection cavity. The dura was closed with interrupted Vicryl, and a piece of Gelfoam was placed with the bone flap replaced with multiple titanium plates and screws. We then located where our right temporal craniotomy would be located. We opened a small segment of the temporalis muscle and fascia with careful attention to keeping it still attached at the superotemporal line. Cerebellar was used to retract the temporalis muscle. We made three bur holes around our entry point centered on the superior temporal gyrus. The dura was opened in a cruciate manner. We made a small corticectomy with bipolar cautery and sharp dissection and entered the superotemporal gyrus and followed directly, staying in normal white matter until we found ourselves on top of the cavernous malformation. This was carefully dissected in all directions and removed. A small bit of hemosiderin-stained tissue was also removed. The operating microscope was then brought in for the case. Using the operating microscope for microdissection, we were able to carefully evaluate all of the walls, which looked like normal white matter or pia in all directions with no evidence of persistent hemosiderin staining or cavernous malformation. The dura was then closed with interrupted Nurolon supplemented with a piece of onlay pericranium and Gelfoam, and then the bone flap was replaced with multiple titanium plates and screws. The temporalis muscle was closed with interrupted Vicryl in the fascia for a watertight closure. The wound was vigorously irrigated with antibiotic and saline and closed with interrupted Vicryl in the galea and then running Monocryl suture in the skin. This was covered with antibiotic ointment and dressed per protocol. The patient remained hemodynamically throughout the surgery. Of note, I, James Johnston, was present for and performed or assisted with the entirety of the procedure. Additionally, no qualified resident was available to assist me. Dr. Feldman assisted me with the initial opening of both craniotomies and resection of cavernous malformations as well as final closure.

Postsurgical Labs

- Patient was taken to ICU following dual craniotomy
- Arterial line placed with all values within normal range
- Urinary catheter placed
- Prothrombin time: 12.7 (normal range 12.1–14.6)
- CBC with differential: all values within normal ranges
- Fluid balance panel: normal values for all except potassium, which was low at 3.4 (normal 3.5–5.1)

mmol/L; chloride, which was high at 108 (normal 98–107) mmol/L; and glucose, which was high at 108 (normal 70–105) mg/dL

- Postsurgical: nausea, vomiting, and severe headache. Oral medications ordered were changed to IV route until PO could be tolerated.

Blood (Arterial)		Normal Range	Unit
Blood Gas Electrolyte and Metabolite (Collected on December 13, 2023, 10:28 AM)			
PH	7.48	7.35–7.45	
PCO2	28	35–45	mmHg
PO2	101	80–100	mmHg
$HCO3^-$	20.8	21–28	mmol/L
Base Deficit	2		
Saturated	98	95–98	%
Total CO2 Arterial	22	22–28	mmol/L
Sodium	135	134–143	mmol/L
Potassium	5.3	3.3–4.6	mmol/L
Ionized Calcium	1.1	1.12–1.30	mmol/L
Glucose	127	70–126	mg/dL
Lactate	2.17	0.7–2.1	mmol/L
Chloride	104	96–109	mmol/L
Creatinine	0.8	0.7–1.5	mg/dL
Hematocrit	40	37–49	%
Hemoglobin	13.5	13–16	g/dL
Blood Electrolyte and Metabolite (Collected on December 14, 2023, 3:55 AM)			
Sodium	139	136–145	mmol/L
Potassium	3.4	3.5–5.1	mmol/L
Chloride	108	98–107	mmol/L
CO2	25	22–29	mmol/L
Anion Gap	6	9–18	mmol/L

Blood (Arterial)		Normal Range	Unit
Glucose	108	70–105	mg/dL
BUN	14	9–21	mg/dL
Creatinine	0.65	0.73–1.18	mg/dL
Calcium	8	8.4–10.2	mg/dL

Urinalysis (Collected on December 13, 2023, 7:55 AM)

Urine (Catheter)		Normal Range	Unit
Urobilinogen	<2	0.2–1	mg/dL
Color	Yellow		
Clarity	Hazy		
pH	7	4.5–8	
Protein	negative		
Glucose	negative		
Ketones	negative		
Bilirubin	negative		
Blood	negative		
Leukocyte Esterase	negative		
Nitrite	negative		
Ascorbic Acid	negative		
Specific Gravity	1.023	1.003–1.030	

Postsurgical MRI was done on December 14, 2023, and compared to the October 2023 scan. Overall interpretation of the scan indicated that the cavernomas were successfully removed as well as the surrounding damaged brain tissue.

Findings

- Status post-right-sided craniotomy for cavernoma resection
- Small heterogenous, proteinaceous fluid–filled surgical cavities within right frontal and right temporal lobes as expected following cavernomas resection
- No acute infarction, intraparenchymal hemorrhage, mass, or mass effect
- Normal morphology of the pituitary–hypothalamic axis
- Expected thin linear dural enhancement adjacent to craniotomy site
- Small pneumocephalus/gas bubbles within intercranial compartment as expected, measuring 5 mm in thickness, associated with minimal local mass effect
- Follow up with neurosurgeon and neurologist to monitor for 9 months post-surgery.
- Goal is to have full cessation of medications. The decrease of medications will begin 9 months post-surgery, which is September 2024.
- No episodes/No issues post-surgery

Current Patient Status

- Follow up with neurosurgeon 2 weeks post-op and 3 months post-op; scheduled for 8 months post-op.
- Follow up with neurologist 1-month post-op and 3 months post-op; scheduled for 9 months post-op.
- 9 months post-op plan to begin slow decrease of medications with desired goal of cessation by December 2025

Chapter 15

Infectious Disease: Case 1

Onset	The patient is an 82-days-old male. He presented to the hospital with a complaint of coughing.
Location	Left temporal skull fracture and a cut on the left leg
Duration	The patient is coughing for a few days
Characteristic	
Alleviating Factors	
Aggravating Factors	
Timing	A diagnosis of bronchopneumonia was made on 03/26/2024
Severity	light

Medical History: The patient is a premature baby (two months earlier than due date).

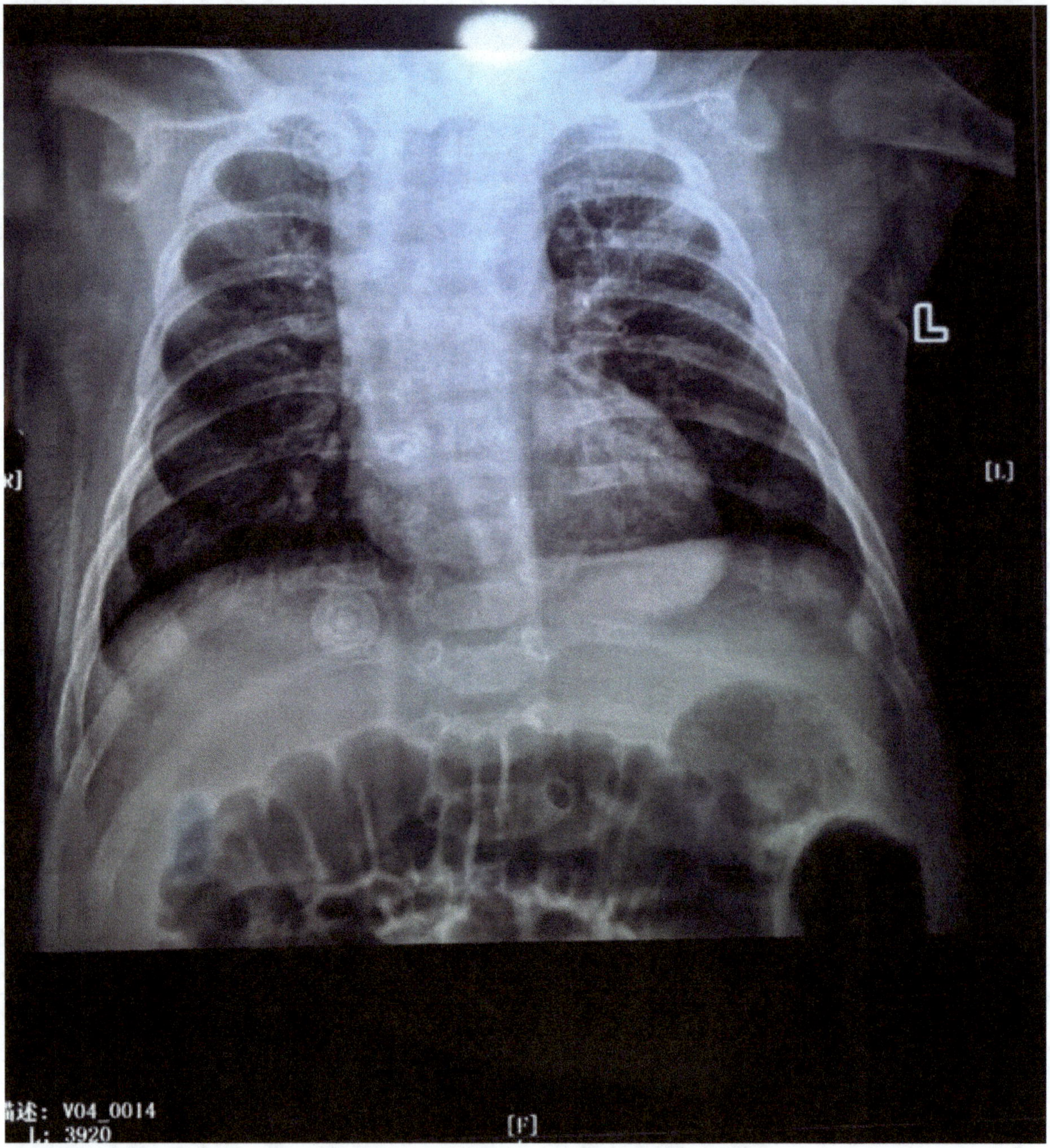

Figure 15.1 Chest X-Ray

- White blood cell count: 12.28 X 10^9/L; Neutrophil count: 16.2%; Lymphocyte: 72.4%; Red blood cell count: 3.7 x 10^12/L; Hemoglobin: 103g/L; Platelets: 389 x 10^9/L; CRP: <6.0mg/L; Ultrasensitive CRP: 1.15 mg/L (↑); Iron: 7.84umol/L (↓)
- Liver and kidney function: No abnormal findings
- Urine and feces tests: No abnormal findings
- Throat swab culture: Negative

Differential Diagnosis

- Pneumonia
- Viral pneumonia
- Mycoplasma pneumonia

Treatment

- Amoxicillin and clavulanate potassium (0.18 g IV)
- Ambroxine (7.5 ng IV) for removing sputum.
- Nebulization with budesonide, terbutaline, acetylcysteine

Chapter 16

Digestive System: Case 2

Onset	The patient is a 22-year-old female. She was diagnosed Celiac disease at the age of 14.
Location	The pain is located in the middle lower region of the abdomen.
Duration	After gluten-containing food is ingested, the symptoms last from 3 days to 1 week.
Characteristic	Stabbing pain in stomach, nausea, diarrhea, vomiting, fatigue, weakness, brain fog, constipation, and muscle pain
Alleviating Factors	Mint, rest, and warm compress
Aggravating Factors	Consumption of gluten, fatty meals, and spicy food
Timing	
Severity	Severe

Physical Examination

- Bloating of abdomen
- Weight loss
- Nonspecific bone or joint pain
- Pale or fatigued appearance

Step 1: What is the most probable diagnosis?

- Celiac Disease/Food allergy
- Irritable bowel syndrome
- Infection

- Ulcerative colitis

Step 2: Based on the patient's medical history, what diagnostic tests should you order?

- Blood Test (tTG-IgA and tTG-G test)
- Tissue Transglutaminase IgA (tTG-IgA) and IgG (tTG-G) are used to help diagnose celiac disease
- Intestinal and Skin Biopsy (inflammation and damage visible under microscope)
- Genetic Testing (human leukocyte antigen (HLA) DQ2 and DQ8)

Step 3: Based on the information on the patient presentation, diagnostic tests, and medical history, what is your decision regarding treating the patient? Why?

- Corticosteroids to relieve inflammation
- Dietary supplements and vitamins
- Gluten-free diet
- Support groups

Chapter 17

Cardiovascular System: Case 3

Onset	The patient is a 76-year-old male. He passed out in the backyard in October 2017 around 5 p.m. and was brought to the hospital by ambulance.
Location	Chest pain
Duration	1 hour
Characteristic	Chest pain, sweating; felt nausea, dizziness, and fatigue, and memory loss
Alleviating Factors	Aspirin/fibrinolytics to reduce blood clotting; oxygen therapy; pain medication
Aggravating Factors	Smoking, overactivity
Timing	
Severity	8/10

The patient has a military background.

The patient has a history of prostate cancer. He had a stent placed in the left groin due to narrow arteries. He has a smoking history and often passes out. At the same time, he feels a shortness of breath.

Patient has flatlined on the ECG four times and was shocked four times before stabilized. A pacemaker was placed.

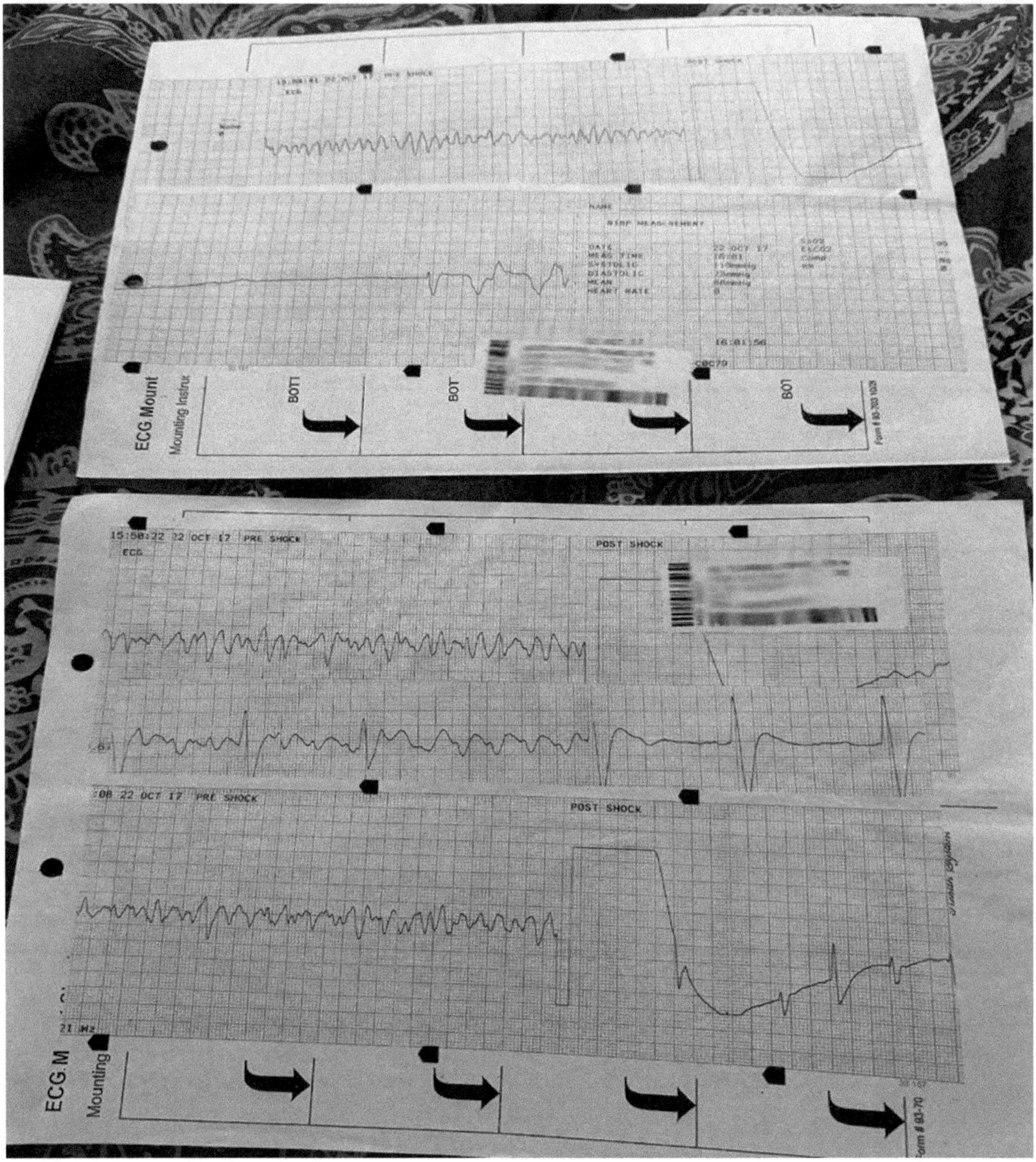

Figure 17.1 ECG

Step 1: What is the most likely diagnosis?

Step 2: Based on the medical history, what diagnostic tests should you order?

- MRI

- ECG,
- Blood Lab Tests
- Chest X-Ray

Step 3: Based on the information from the patient presentation, diagnostic tests, and medical history, what is your decision regarding treating the patient? Why?

The patient had an emergency quadruple bypass to reroute blood flow in the heart. The life expectancy after surgery is 18 to 20 years.

After surgery, clopidogrel bisulfate 75 mg (1 tablet/day), amiodarone 200 mg (twice/day), aspirin 81 mg/day, iron polysaccharide 150 oral capsule (1 capsule/day), pravastatin 20mg (1 tablet/day), and Warfarin 5 mg (1 tablet/day)

Post-operation orders:

- Clean wound daily (wash gently with soap and water)
- Do not swim or take baths
- Do not use lotions or creams

Medical Information

Order Name	Order Details
Activity Level Post Discharge	Increase activity gradually
Activity Level Post Discharge	No sitting in front seat for 4 weeks; or cleared by your physician
Activity Level Post Discharge	No lifting greater than 10 lbs for 2 months
Activity Level Post Discharge	Weigh yourself daily at the same time and on the same scale
Activity Level Post Discharge	Elevate legs when sitting
Diet Post Discharge	Cardiac diet
Discharge Diagnostic Exams	07-Nov-2017 12:43:00 EST, PALAT Chest Xray at Medical Office Building on postop visit with surgeon
Special Discharge Instructions	07-Nov-2017 12:43:00 EST, Orders for Skill Nursing Facility: Sliding scale insulin coverage qAC and qHS if patient is diabetic
Special Discharge Instructions	07-Nov-2017 12:43:00 EST, Orders for Skilled Nursing Facility: Incentive spirometry 20 times per hour
Special Discharge Instructions	07-Nov-2017 12:43:00 EST, Orders for Skilled Nursing Facility:

Out of bed to chair during the day. Cardiac reclining chair in

room at all times

Special Discharge Instructions 07-Nov-2017 12:43:00 EST, Orders for Skilled Nursing Facility:

Notify surgeon with changes in patient's medication profile

Special Discharge Instructions 07-Nov-2017 12:43:00 EST, Orders for Skilled Nursing Facility:

Notify surgeon when patient arrives to skilled nursing facility

Special Discharge Instructions 07-Nov-2017 12:43:00 EST, Orders for Skilled Nursing Facility:

Notify surgeon if patient's temperature >38 C, heart rate > 120

or <30, blood pressure > 160 mmHg

Special Discharge Instructions 07-Nov-2017 12:43:00 EST, Orders for Skilled Nursing Facility:

Shower daily in the morning with antibacterial soap

Special Discharge Instructions 07-Nov-2017 12:43:00 EST, Incision care. Monitor for signs of

Infection and bleeding and notify surgeon with any changes.

Special Discharge Instructions 07-Nov-2017 12:43:00 EST, Daily incisional site dressing

Change with betadine and gauze dressing with paper tape after

morning shower

Special Discharge Instructions 07-Nov-2017 12:43:00 EST, Check blood sugar qAC and qHS if

patient is diabetic

Special Discharge Instructions 07-Nov-2017 12:43:00 EST, Notify Physician of weight gain 2

pounds overnight or 5 pounds in one week

Special Discharge Instructions 07-Nov-2017 12:43:00 EST, Notify Physician if symptoms of

heart failure are present

Special Discharge Instructions 07-Nov-2017 12:43:00 EST, Notify Physician if you experience

	shortness of breath at rest or with minimal activity
Special Discharge Instructions	07-Nov-2017 12:43:00 EST, Notify Physician if you experience
	increased swelling of legs

Diet order: cardiac diet; low-fat and low-sodium items free of salt and pepper; limit alcohol intake

Vegetables	**Serving Size**	
Anchovies, fillets	1 each	Low
Asparagus, cooked	5 spears	Medium
Asparagus, raw	5 spears	Medium
Beans, green, cooked	1 cup	Medium
Beets, cooked, sliced	1 cup	Low
Broccoli, cooked, chopped	1 cup	High
Broccoli, raw, chopped	1 cup	High
Brussels sprouts, cooked	1 cup	High
Brussels sprouts, raw	1 cup	High
Cabbage, Chinese, raw, shredded	1 cup	Medium
Cabbage, napa, raw, shredded	1 cup	High
Cabbage, red, raw, shredded	1 cup	Medium
Carrots, cooked, slices	1 cup	Medium
Carrots, raw, strips or slices	1 cup	Low
Cauliflower, cooked	1 cup	Medium
Cauliflower, raw	1 cup	Low
Celery	1 stalk	Low
Collard Greens, cooked	1 cup	High
Corn, yellow, cooked	1 cup	Low
Corn, yellow, raw	1 cup	Low
Cucumber	1 medium	Low
Eggplant, cooked, cubed	1 cup	Low

Vegetables	Serving Size	
Eggplant, raw, cubed	1 cup	Low
Endive, raw, chopped	1 cup	High
Fennel	1 bulb	Low
Garlic	3 cloves	Low
Kale, raw, chopped	1 cup	High
Leek, raw	1 medium	High
Lettuce, arugula	½ cup	Low
Lettuce, Boston/Bibb, raw	1 cup	High
Lettuce, green leaf, raw	1 cup	High
Lettuce, iceberg, raw	1 cup	Low
Lettuce, red leaf, raw	1 cup	Medium
Lettuce, Romaine, raw	1 cup	High
Mushrooms, raw	1 cup	Low
Mustard greens, raw, chopped	1 cup	High
Okra, cooked	1 cup	High
Onions, green/scallions, raw	1 cup	High
Onions, white/red/yellow, raw	1 cup	Low
Parsley, raw	1 cup	High
Parsnips, cooked	1 cup	Low
Peas & Onions, frozen, cooked	1 cup	Medium
Peas, green, cooked	1 cup	High
Peas, green, frozen, cooked	10 oz	High
Peas, sugar snap, cooked	1 cup	High

Vegetables	Serving Size	
Pepper, green bell	1 medium	Low
Pepper, jalapeno	1 medium	Low
Pepper, red bell	1 medium	Low
Pepper, red chili, hot	1 each	Low
Pepper, yellow sweet	1 medium	Low
Potato, red, cooked	1 medium	Low
Potato, sweet, cooked	1 medium	Low
Potato, white, baked	1 medium	Low
Shallots, chopped	1 Tbsp	Low
Snow peas, raw	1 cup	Low
Spaghetti/marinara sauce	1 cup	Medium
Spinach, cooked	1 cup	High
Spinach, frozen	10 oz.	High
Spinach, raw	1 cup	High
Squash, acorn	1 cup	Low
Squash, butternut, cooked, cubed	1 cup	Low
Squash, summer, cooked	1 cup	Low
Swiss Chard, raw	1 cup	High
Tomato paste	1 Tbsp	Low
Tomato sauce, canned, no salt	1 cup	Low
Tomato, plum	1	Low
Tomato, raw	1 medium	Low

Vegetables	Serving Size	
Tomatoes, canned, whole	1 cup	Low
Tomatoes, cherry	1 cup	Low
Tomatoes, sun-dried	1 cup	Medium

Follow-Up

The patient has a better diet. He has passed out twice since the surgery and has annual checkups.

Chapter 18

HEENT: Case 1

Onset	The patient is a 23-year-old female who noticed vision changes and experienced itchy, red, and stinging eyes in May 2023. Moreover, astigmatism and myopia were noted.
Location	Cornea of eye
Duration	Lasting a few hours and occurring every week or every two weeks
Characteristic	Itchy eyes, red eyes, stinging/burning eyes, astigmatism, loss of vision
Alleviating Factors	Use of antibiotics (maxifloxacin) and steroids (difluprednate)
Aggravating Factors	Bright light or direct sunlight irritates
Timing	Symptoms are intermittent
Severity	Mild

LASIK surgery is eye surgery that reshapes the cornea to correct vision; however, a rare complication like post-LASIK ectasia can arise, leading to further vision issues.

Medical History

The patient had no prior use of contact lenses. The patient has no history of cardiovascular disease, high blood pressure, cataracts, or mental illness. The patient started wearing glasses at very young age. In her mid-teen, she began developing styes. In 2015, the patient had signs of chalazions. A chalazion, also known as a meibomian cyst, is a red, firm, painless nodule on the eyelid that results from a blocked oil gland. The patient had LASIK surgery in 2020 after the chalazion was removed. Another surgical removal of a chalazion was conducted in 2022. Complications with LASIK surgery started in 2023.

Physical Examination

- Bulging of the eye, intermittent pain
- Initial findings from an optometrist: abnormal appearance of the corneas, cloudiness on the exterior part of the cornea, protruding blood vessels
- An ophthalmologist found thinning of the cornea and change of shape.

Step 1: What is the possible diagnosis?

Step 2: Based on the medical history, what diagnostic tests should you order?

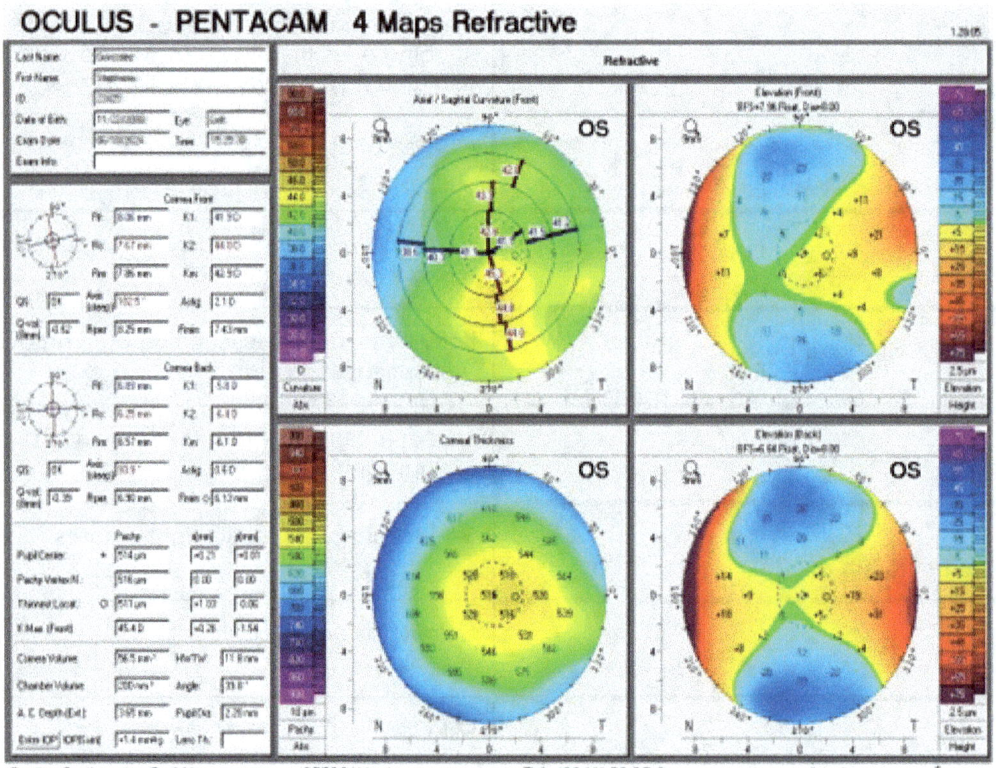

Figure 18.1a Tomography OS

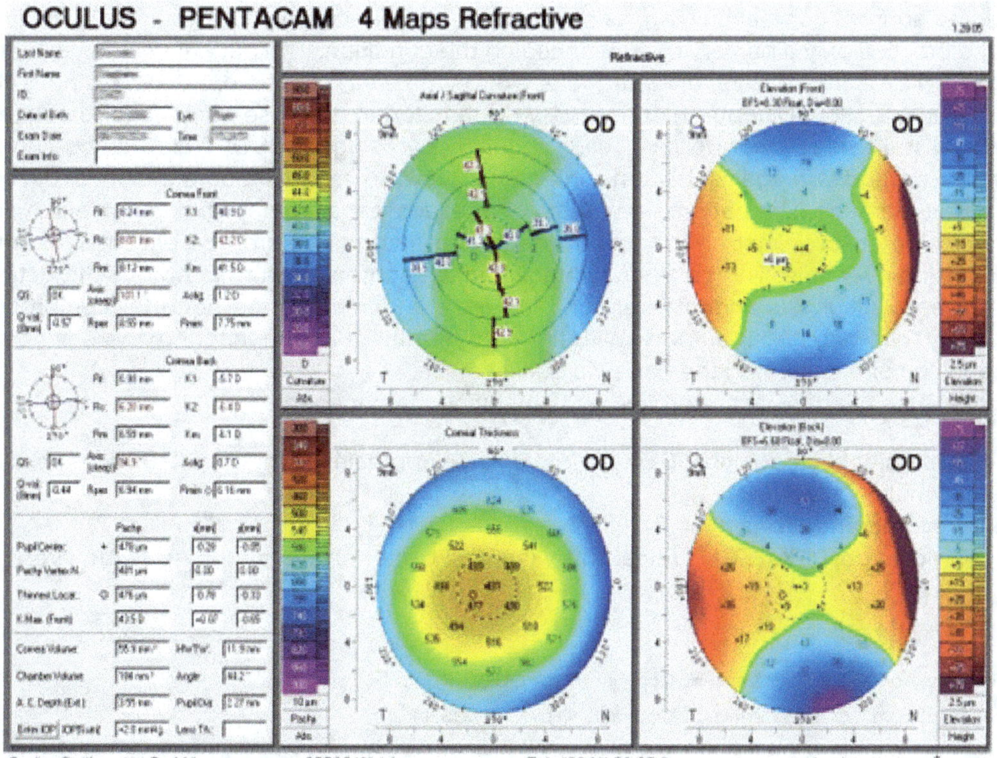

Figure 18.1b Tomography OD

Figures 18.1a and 18.1b show a 3D image of the cornea. The image assesses the entire cornea: anterior and posterior surfaces. There are two images, one for each eye. Warm colors such as red, orange, and yellow indicate thinness of the cornea. Cool colors such as green, blue, and purple indicate thickness of cornea. Based on this assessment the doctor noticed an abnormal thinness and change in shape of the cornea in both eyes. If you look at the imaging for corneal thickness of the left eye in the lower left quadrant of Figure 18.1a, you notice the numbers in the center are in the low 500s, while the corneal thickness of the right eye, shown in the lower left quadrant of Figure 18.1b, is in the high 400s. This indicates that corneal thinness of the left eye was slightly higher than in the right. The higher the number, the worse the condition. Now, if you look at the Elevation front and back images for both eyes, you will notice there are warm colors on the sides of the corneas. That indicates not only a thin cornea but also one that has begun to change shape. A normal cornea should be round like a basketball. These are more almond shaped.

The patient is developing post-LASIK ectasia. Post-LASIK ectasia is a rare complication of LASIK eye surgery, causing the cornea to lose its shape and bulge forward. This leads to distorted vision, often necessitating corrective lenses. It occurs in less than 1% of the population who have had laser surgery and is more likely to occur in patients with inherently weak or thin corneas or those with mild keratoconus. Normally, there is a constant flow of fluid that creates pressure on the inside structures of the eye; when a thin spot develops on the cornea, eye pressure will cause it to flex outwards.

Currently, the severity of her condition is mild. If progression of the disease occurs, it could lead to bulging of the eye, double vision, halos around lights, and worsening of vision. These symptoms are indicative of the structural changes occurring in the cornea. Preventive measures were taken to slow down or halt the progression of LASIK ectasia.

Step 3: Based on the information on the patient presentation, diagnostic tests, medical history, what is your decision to treat the patient? Why?

The treatment plan for this patient includes several key components. In severe cases, surgery might be necessary to address corneal bulging; as of now, that is not necessary for this patient. Medications and good hygiene practice play a primary role in managing the condition. The patient was prescribed an antibiotic like moxifloxacin and a steroid, difluprednate, along with erythromycin ophthalmic ointment to control inflammation and infection. Difluprednate is a very strong steroid; overuse could lead to cataracts, so the patient was advised to clean her upper eyelids regularly by using OCuSOFT Lid Scrubs and BRIOTECH Topical Spray to defend skin against bacterial infections. It is also crucial that the patient avoid eye rubbing to prevent further damage. The patient now wears glasses to treat astigmatism and myopia. A comprehensive treatment plan ensures that all aspects of the patient's condition are addressed, aiming to stabilize and improve vision over time. This case study highlights the complex nature of post-LASIK ectasia and the importance of early diagnosis and intervention. The case underscores the need for comprehensive eye care, particularly following LASIK surgery. With the right treatment and monitoring, there is hope for stabilizing the condition and improving the patient's quality of life.

Medication: use of antibiotics, steroids, and anti-inflammatory agents

- Moxifloxacin ophthalmic solution (0.5%); difulprednate ophthalmic emulsion (0.05%); erythromycin ophthalmic ointment

  Hygiene recommendations:
- OCuSOFT lid scrub; BRIOTECH topical spray (against bacteria); avoid rubbing of the eyes

Image Credits

Fig. 18.1a: Screenshot from OCULUS Pentacam. Copyright © by OCULUS, Inc.

Fig. 18.1b: Screenshot from OCULUS Pentacam. Copyright © by OCULUS, Inc.

Chapter 19

Musculoskeletal System: Case 2

Onset	The patient is a 66-year-old male. He complained of severe pain in the right lower leg.
Location	It is located deep in the gastrocnemius muscle.
Duration	The pain has lasted for more than 1 hour.
Characteristic	No radiation; constant
Alleviating Factors	None
Aggravating Factors	
Timing	The pain started in the early afternoon and got worse after dinner.
Severity	8/10

Background: The patient spent 1 week in Orlando, Florida, with his family (from Christmas to the new year of 2023). He and his wife drove to Pensacola on New Year's Day (1/1/2023) and stayed at his nephew's house. His nephew was repairing his house due to the flood damage brought by Hurricane Ian. The patient helped his brother rewire the house and did some other work, such as holding the ladders.

On January 2, 2023, the patient drove to Birmingham, Alabama and visited a friend. They arrived at his friend's home around 2:00 pm. Around 5:00 pm, they went out for dinner and ate pizza and drank some lemonade. The patient felt some pain on his right leg. Around 6:30 pm, the patient felt the pain was getting worse. Local massage did not help, and the severe pain lasted for more than 1 hour.

Social History: He is a traveling medical physician. No smoking; drinks socially.

Medical History: He has hypertension and is on medication now (calcium channel blocker amlodipine).

Vaccine: He received one booster dose of COVID-19 vaccine before Christmas of 2022. He also received his annual flu vaccine then.

Family history: He and his wife have three daughters and one son. His uncle died from colon cancer 2 years ago.

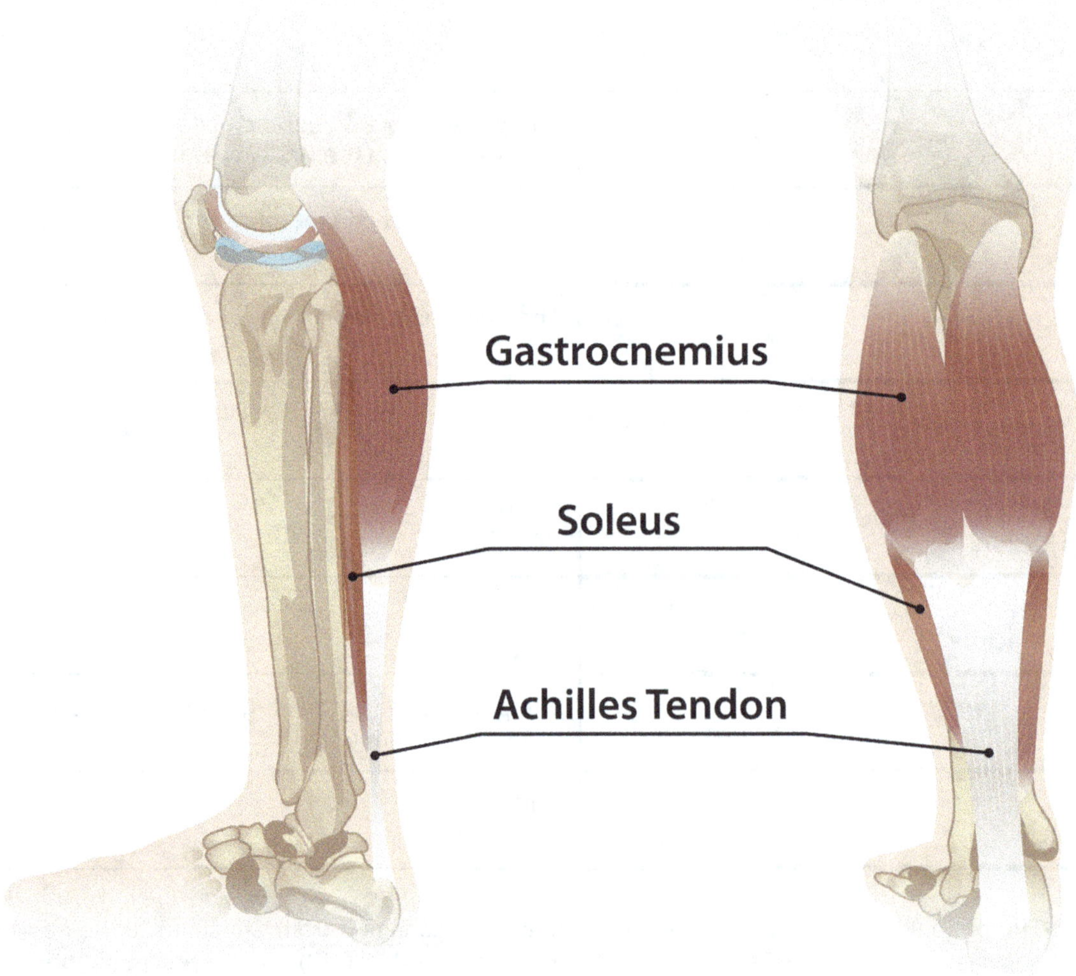

Figure 19.1 Calf Muscle

Step 1: What are the possible diagnoses?

- Deep vein thrombosis
- Strained muscle
- Muscular spasm
- COVID-19

Step 2: Which tests should you order?

- CT
- Doppler ultrasound
- D-dimer

Step 3: How to treat the patient?

- Ibuprofen
- Aspirin

Image Credits

Fig. 19.1: Copyright © 2019 by InjuryMap (CC BY-SA 4.0) at https://commons.wikimedia.org/wiki/File:Lower_leg_muscles.svg.

Chapter 20

Endocrine System: Case 3

Onset	The patient is a 21-year-old female presenting with an intermittent headache. The patient is also complaining of a rash and constant drainage from her bilateral mammary papillae that began in February 2024.
Location	Head Bilateral mammary papillae
Duration	February 2024 to present
Characteristic	Headache: sinus headache Rash: red, itchy, raised, flaky, burning, Galactorrhea: constant milk-like discharge
Alleviating Factors	The patient did not take any medications for her headache. Rash: antibiotics
Aggravating Factors	Headache: none Rash: sweating
Timing	Symptoms are constant but vary in severity. Headache: At first onset, patient experienced a headache twice a week. Currently, she experiences a headache daily, with each episode lasting 30 minutes. Rash: Patient experiences constant drainage and itching.
Severity	Headache: Pain rated as 5/10 Rash: Pain rated as 4/10

The patient reports that her headache was intermittent, occurring about twice a week when her symptoms first began. Currently, she experiences daily headaches with episodes lasting 30 minutes and rates the pain as a 5/10. She reports that the rash is constantly itching and rates the pain as a 4/10. She denies any pain associated with her galactorrhea; however, she states that the drainage is constant.

Galactorrhea: milk or a milk-like discharge from the breast, unrelated to pregnancy or breastfeeding

First Assessment

On July 8th, 2024, the patient was seen by her primary care physician. After conducting a visual examination, the patient was diagnosed with cellulitis (bacterial skin infection) and candidiasis (skin yeast infection) of the chest wall. Patient was placed on Bactrim DS (antibiotic) twice daily (b.i.d.) for 10 days, fluconazole (antifungal) once daily for 7 days, and she was given a nystatin cream (antifungal) to apply externally twice a day (b.i.d.).

Second Assessment

The patient returned on July 23rd, 2024. She reports some improvement to the rash with the antibiotics but is still experiencing constant drainage from her bilateral mammary papillae and daily headaches. Blood tests were ordered, and the patient was found to have elevated levels of prolactin.

CBC With Differential/Platelet

	NAME	VALUE	REFERENCE RANGE
F	WBC	5.1	3.4-10.8 (x10E3/uL)
F	RBC	4.97	3.77-5.28 (x10E6/uL)
F	Hemoglobin	13.7	11.1-15.9 (g/dL)
F	Hematocrit	42.5	34.0-46.6 (%)
F	MCV	86	79-97 (fL)
F	MCH	27.6	26.6-33.0 (pg)
F	MCHC	32.2	31.5-35.7 (g/dL)
F	RDW	12.4	11.7-15.4 (%)
F	Platelets	289	150-450 (x10E3/uL)
F	Neutrophils	45	Not Estab. (%)
F	Lymphs	43	Not Estab. (%)
F	Monocytes	6	Not Estab. (%)
F	Eos	5	Not Estab. (%)
F	Basos	1	Not Estab. (%)
	Immature Cells		
F	Neutrophils (Absolute)	2.3	1.4-7.0 (x10E3/uL)
F	Lymphs (Absolute)	2.2	0.7-3.1 (x10E3/uL)
F	Monocytes(Absolute)	0.3	0.1-0.9 (x10E3/uL)
F	Eos (Absolute)	0.2	0.0-0.4 (x10E3/uL)

F	Baso (Absolute)	0.1	0.0-0.2 (x10E3/uL)
F	Immature Granulocytes	0	Not Estab. (%)
F	Immature Grans (Abs)	0.0	0.0-0.1 (x10E3/uL)
	NRBC		

Comp. Metabolic Panel (14)

	NAME	VALUE	REFERENCE RANGE
F	Glucose	79	70-99 (mg/dL)
F	BUN	10	6-20 (mg/dL)
F	Creatinine	0.92	0.57-1.00 (mg/dL)
F	eGFR	91	>59 (mL/min/1.73)
F	BUN/Creatinine Ratio	11	9-23
F	Sodium	139	134-144 (mmol/L)
F	Potassium	4.8	3.5-5.2 (mmol/L)
F	Chloride	104	96-106 (mmol/L)
F	Carbon Dioxide, Total	21	20-29 (mmol/L)
F	Calcium	9.3	8.7-10.2 (mg/dL)
F	Protein, Total	7.0	6.0-8.5 (g/dL)
F	Albumin	4.2	4.0-5.0 (g/dL)
F	Globulin, Total	2.8	1.5-4.5 (g/dL)
F	Bilirubin, Total	0.2	0.0-1.2 (mg/dL)
F	Alkaline Phosphatase	52	42-106 (IU/L)
F	AST (SGOT)	18	0-40 (IU/L)
F	ALT (SGPT)	13	0-32 (IU/L)

TSH+Free T4

	NAME	VALUE	REFERENCE RANGE
F	TSH	1.020	0.450-4.500 (uIU/mL)
F	T4,Free(Direct)	1.13	0.82-1.77 (ng/dL)

Prolactin

	NAME	VALUE	REFERENCE RANGE
F	Prolactin	34.5	4.8-33.4 (ng/mL)

Figure 20.1e Lab Test Results

Most nonpregnant women have prolactin levels less than 25 ng/mL. Due to the patient's elevated prolactin levels, an MRI of the brain with contrast with special emphasis on the pituitary gland was ordered. An MRI was performed on August 30th, 2024. Patient is found to have a microadenoma.

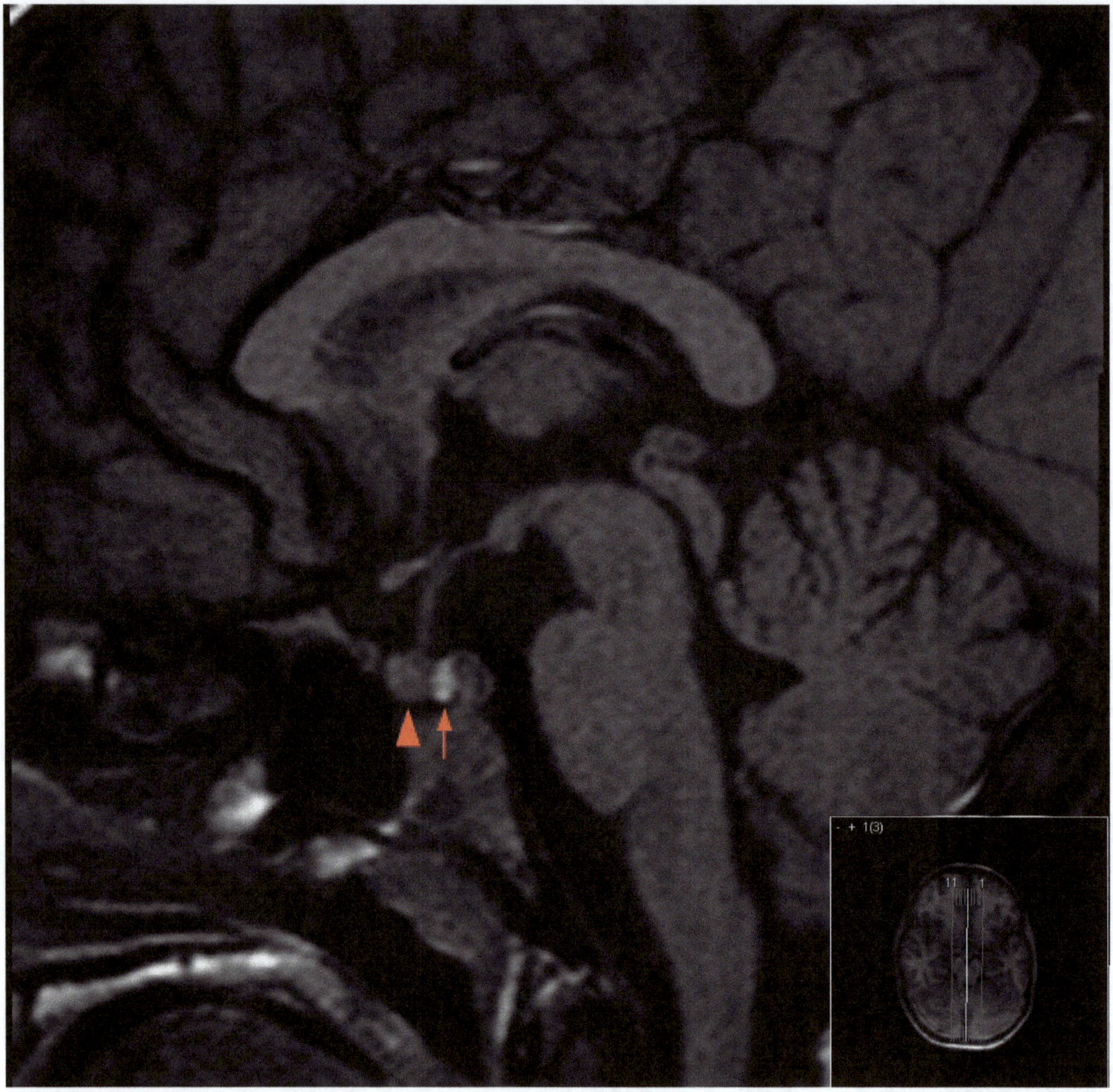

Figure 20.2a Sagitall MRI of the Brain

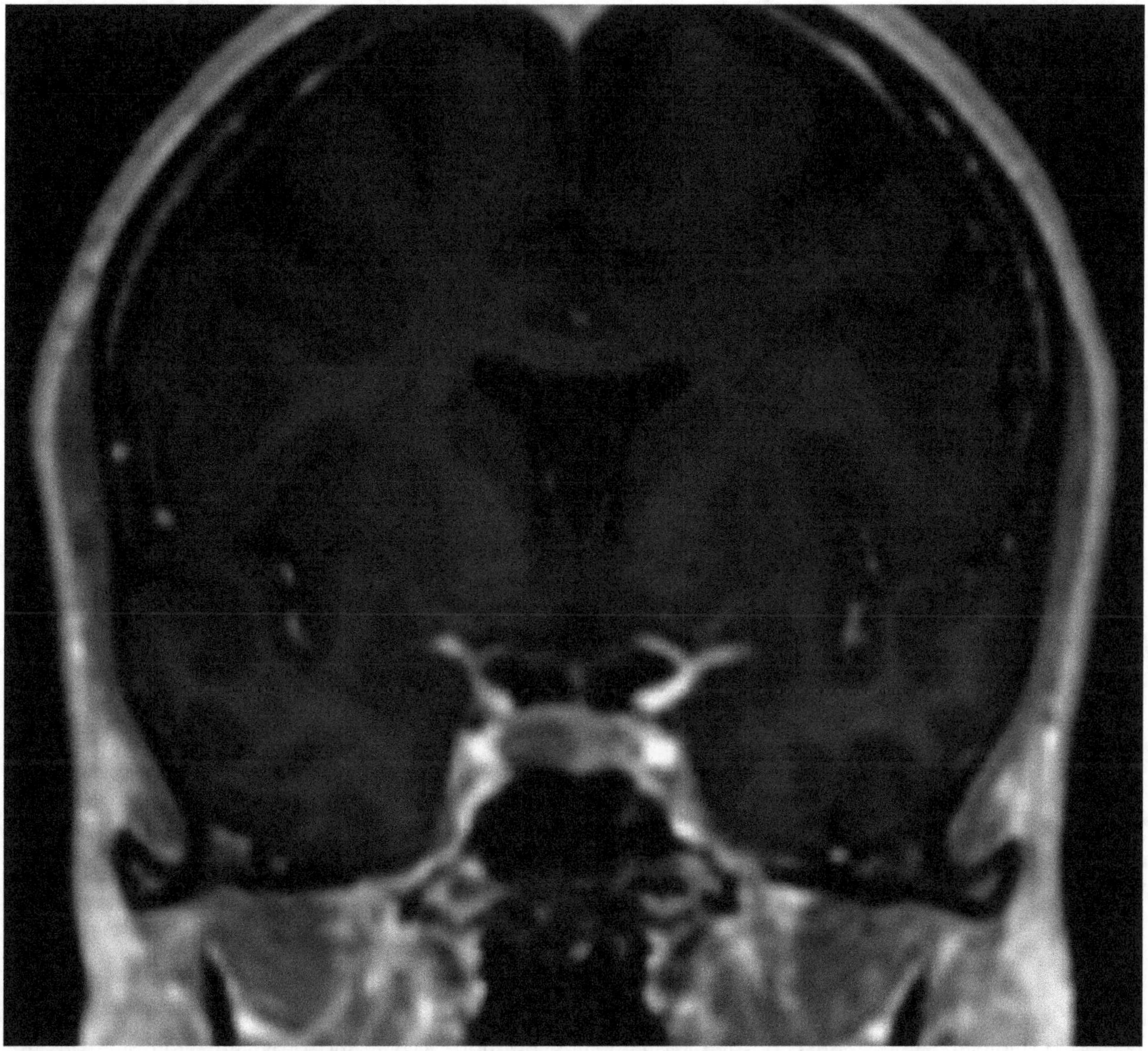

Figure 20.2b Coronal MRI of the Brain

The sagittal plane view of the pituitary shows a darker gray lesion within the pituitary gland (Figure 20.2a). The mass can also be seen by looking at the coronal plane, where the rounded gray lesion is more apparent (Figure 20.2b).

Diagnosis

- Pituitary tumor
- Hypothyroidism
- Breast Cancer

The patient is diagnosed with a functioning pituitary microadenoma (prolactinoma) resulting in hyperprolactinemia. A pituitary microadenoma is a benign tumor of the pituitary gland with a diameter less than

10 mm. As many as 10% of the population may have a microadenoma, but most do not cause symptoms. Microadenomas are categorized as either functioning (hormone-secreting) or non-functioning (non-hormone-secreting).

Prolactinomas are prolactin-producing tumors of the pituitary gland, and account for up to 40% of pituitary adenomas. Excess prolactin production disrupts the hypothalamic–pituitary–gonadal axis, inhibiting gonadotropin-releasing hormone (GnRH).

Prolactinomas have several distinct clinical features in men and women. In men, they lead to several features, such as decreased libido and erectile dysfunction. In women, they lead to amenorrhea (absence of menstruation), galactorrhea, and infertility.

Prolactin is secreted by lactotroph cells in the anterior pituitary gland. For males, it supports testosterone and sexual function. For females, it functions with breast development and milk production. The secretion of prolactin is regulated by two main hormones: thyrotropin-releasing hormone (TRH) and dopamine.

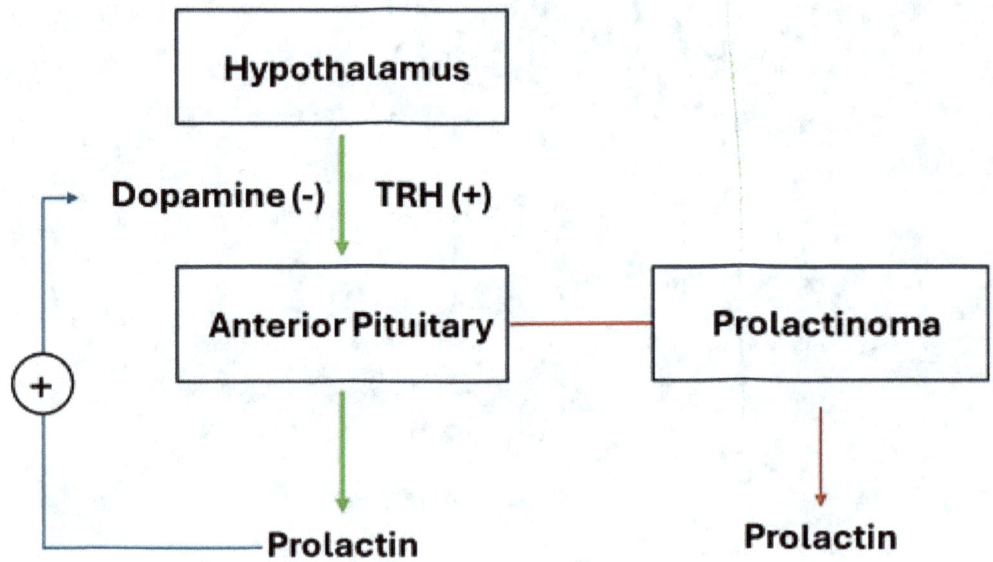

Figure 20.3 Regulation Pathways for Prolactin

TRH stimulates the release of thyroid-stimulating hormone (TSH) and prolactin. TRH acts on TRH receptors in lactotroph cells, which produce prolactin. Conditions like primary hypothyroidism, which can increase TRH levels, then cause an elevated prolactin level.

Treatment

Patient will see a specialist in April 2025. The likely treatment is a dopamine agonist, which will reduce prolactin production and shrink the tumor. The first-choice medication is cabergoline.

Cabergoline is a pharmaceutical drug commonly used to treat hyperprolactinemic-related conditions such as prolactinoma. It is a dopamine agonist with high affinity for dopamine receptors (D2R). It binds to the D2R on lactotrophs, or prolactin cells, of the anterior pituitary gland to inhibit the production and secretion of prolactin. It can shrink tumors, normalize prolactin (PRL) levels, and restore the negative feedback mechanism within the hypothalamic–pituitary axis.

Image Credits

Fig. 20.1a-e: Copyright © by Labcorp | Birmingham.

Fig. 20.2a: Copyright © 2010 by Hellerhoff (CC BY-SA 4.0) at https://commons.wikimedia.org/wiki/File:Hypophyse_MRT_sag.png.

Fig. 20.2b: Copyright © 2009 by Hellerhoff (CC BY-SA 3.0) at https://commons.wikimedia.org/wiki/File:Cavum_septi_pellucidi_MRT_cor_T1.jpg.

Chapter 21

Digestive System: Case 3

Onset	A 22-year-old female complains of fatigue, chronic migraines, shortness of breath, abdominal pain, chest pain, and gastrointestinal discomfort that started at the beginning of 2023.
Location	
Duration	From the beginning of 2023 to present
Characteristic	
Alleviating Factors	
Aggravating Factors	
Timing	
Severity	Fatigue: severe

Medical history: Prior to the onset of symptoms, patient had a history of Helicobacter pylori infection, which was confirmed with endoscopy.

Family history: diabetes, rheumatoid arthritis, hypertension, and breast cancer

Social history: no smoking or drinking

Diet: dairy-free diet and no red meats (pork, beef, or lamb)

Current Medications: Tylenol for migraines

Differential Diagnosis:

1. Iron deficiency anemia
2. Irritable bowel syndrome
3. Gastritis
4. Peptic ulcer

Tests Ordered

A complete blood count, basic metabolic panel, echocardiogram, vitamin blood test panel, brain MRI, gluten sensitivity test, and cortisol and C-reactive protein tests.

The CBC, BMP, and vitamin blood test panel would allow for confirmation or ruling out of iron deficiency or other vitamin or mineral deficiencies. The echocardiogram was used to rule out any heart issues that may have led to the symptoms of chest pain and shortness of breath. A brain MRI was suggested to rule out the possibility of a complication in the patient's brain causing her migraines, brain fog, and fatigue. The gluten sensitivity, cortisol, and CRP tests were done to assess whether the GI symptoms were being caused by an allergy, stress, inflammation, infection, or other causes.

- First, the**CBC**revealed abnormalities in several areas, including iron binding capacity and essential vitamins like C, B6, B2, B1, and B12, as well as minerals such as magnesium, zinc, and ferritin. These deficiencies suggest possible nutritional issues or absorption problems that could be impacting overall health.
- TheBMP, or **basic metabolic panel**, came back normal
- **Gluten sensitivity** is elevated, which points towards a possible gluten intolerance or sensitivity that could be influencing symptoms.
- **Brain MRI**showed mineral deposition in the medial basal ganglia. No mass was detected
- **Echocardiogram**detected tricuspid valve regurgitation.
- Lastly,**cortisol and CRPlevels** were both elevated, which suggests an inflammatory or stress response, possibly tying into other symptoms the patient is experiencing.

Findings

Brain/intracranial contents: There is a subtle increased T1-weighted signal projected along the medial basal ganglia in a fairly symmetric fashion that is nonspecific, though it may be seen with mineral deposition and has been described with hepatic dysfunction. There is somewhat more extensive adjacent decreased signal on the susceptibility-weighted imaging, which may also be seen with mineral deposition. No significant edema or enhancement is seen at within these regions.

The brain otherwise appears to demonstrate appropriate signal characteristics. The diffusion imaging reveals no evidence of recent infarction. The ventricular system is within normal limits in size configuration. No extra-axial fluid collection or significant mass effect is identified.

- Craniocervical Junction/C1-2: No significant abnormality
- Vascular Flow-Voids: No significant abnormality
- Orbits: No significant abnormality of visualized orbits.
- Sinuses/Mastoids: No significant abnormality.
- Additional Findings: None.

Impressions

- Normal left ventricular size and systolic function.
- Normal diastolic function.
- Mild tricuspid regurgitation.

Findings (Part Two)

- Left Ventricle: LV chamber size is normal. LV wall thickness is normal. The estimated left ventricle ejection fraction is 65%–70% (normal). Normal left atrial pressure and diastolic function. LV relaxation is normal. Mitral E/A: 1.53. Average E/E': 4.56. Peak TR V: 2.66 m/s.
- Right Ventricle: RV size is normal
- Left Atrium: LA chamber size is normal.
- Right Atrium: RA chamber size is normal.
- Aortic Valve: The mitral valve is structurally normal. There is no aortic regurgitation. There is no aortic valve stenosis.
- Mitral Valve: The mitral valve is structurally normal. There is no aortic regurgitation. There is no mitral stenosis.
- Tricuspid Valve: Tricuspid valve is structurally normal. There is mild tricuspid regurgitation. Estimated RVSP systolic pressure is 31.33 mmHg. TV regurgitation peak velocity: 2.66 m/s. Right atrial pressure is 3 mmHg.
- Pulmonary Valve: The pulmonic valve appears grossly normal. There is no pulmonic regurgitation.
- Pericardium: The pericardium is normal.
- Aorta: The aortic root, ascending aorta, descending aorta, and aortic arch are all within normal limits. The portion of the abdominal aorta visualized appears normal in size.
- Venous: IVC diameter is 0.98 cm. The IVC is not dilated and collapses >50% with inspiration. (RAP: 5mmHg).
- Thrombus/Mass: There is no intracardiac mass or thrombus identified.

Iron and Total Iron Binding Capacity			**Normal Range**	**Unit**
	Iron Total	141	40–190	mcg/dL
	Iron Binding Capacity	551	250–450	mcg/dL
	% Saturation	26	16–45	%
Ferritin		5	16–154	ng/mL
Cortisol, Total, LC/MS		28.3	4.6-20.6 (8–10 AM); 1.8–13.6 (4–6 PM)	mcg/dL
HS CRP		2.6	<1.0	mg/L

All lab tests are done with a fasting blood sample.

There are also deficiencies in several vitamins and minerals such as vitamin C, B6, B2, B1, B12, magnesium and zinc.

A high cortisol level could indicate chronic stress within the body and could be due to infection, nutrient deficiencies, inflammation, food sensitivity, and blood sugar imbalances. A high CRP value could coincide with a high cortisol level indicating recent infection and inflammation within the body. High CRP values are associated with inflammatory bowel disease, rheumatoid arthritis, lupus, pancreatitis, and respiratory infections.

Diagnosis

Based on lab work findings, it was confirmed that the patient has iron deficiency anemia (low ferritin levels and high iron binding capacity). The symptoms listed earlier also coincide with symptoms associated with anemia (dizziness, brain fog, fatigue). The gluten allergy was shown from the allergy test as well as low vitamin levels from the panel conducted. This case is still ongoing and does not have a definite overall diagnosis, but based on symptoms and tests done, we can conclude that the patient most likely suffers from celiac disease or other known gastrointestinal disorders. A celiac disease diagnosis is possible due to the gluten allergy test and the patient being deficient in vitamins and iron. The patient eating gluten without knowing that it was an allergen could have led to the gradual destruction of the small intestine's lining and essential vitamins obtained from the diet to not be absorbed.

Treatment

This includes iron supplements, a gluten-free diet, vitamin supplements, and atenolol for migraines.

Follow-Up

Some recommendations include continuing a gluten-free diet, testing again in 6 months to see whether labs are normal, following up with doctor to see whether the treatment is working or changes need to be made, and calling the doctor if symptoms worsen or do not improve after 3 months.

Chapter 22

Reproductive System: Case 2

Onset	The patient is a 48-year-old African American female. During her routine mammogram screening, a nodule was found in her right breast. A biopsy from her right breast as well as the axillary lymph nodes was done on June 14th, 2024.
Location	Right breast
Duration	
Characteristic	Malignant PR (+), ER (+), HER 2 (-)
Alleviating Factors	
Aggravating Factors	
Timing	
Severity	Stage 2 to 3

The patient is from Fort Lauderdale, Florida, and is currently residing in Albany, Georgia.

Family Medical History: None

Past Medical History: Palpitations, type 2 diabetes, asthma, pneumonia, gastrointestinal reflux, anemia, tachycardia, obstructive sleep apnea, hypomagnesia, benign essential hypertension.

The following diagnostic tests were performed: Bone scans, CT scans of the abdomen and pelvis with IV contrast, ultrasounds, and chest X rays.

During the physical examination, the following factors were present:

Many calcifications were scattered throughout the whole breast. The breast tissue was very dense, which made screening difficult. Palpitations were evident, and the scans of the lungs, heart, thyroid, and aorta appeared to be normal. An enlarged node was present in the axillary region.

The patient has lost a significant amount of weight (210lbs to 134lbs). She has fatigue, nausea, and fever. She currently is on oxygen treatment for her respiratory issues.

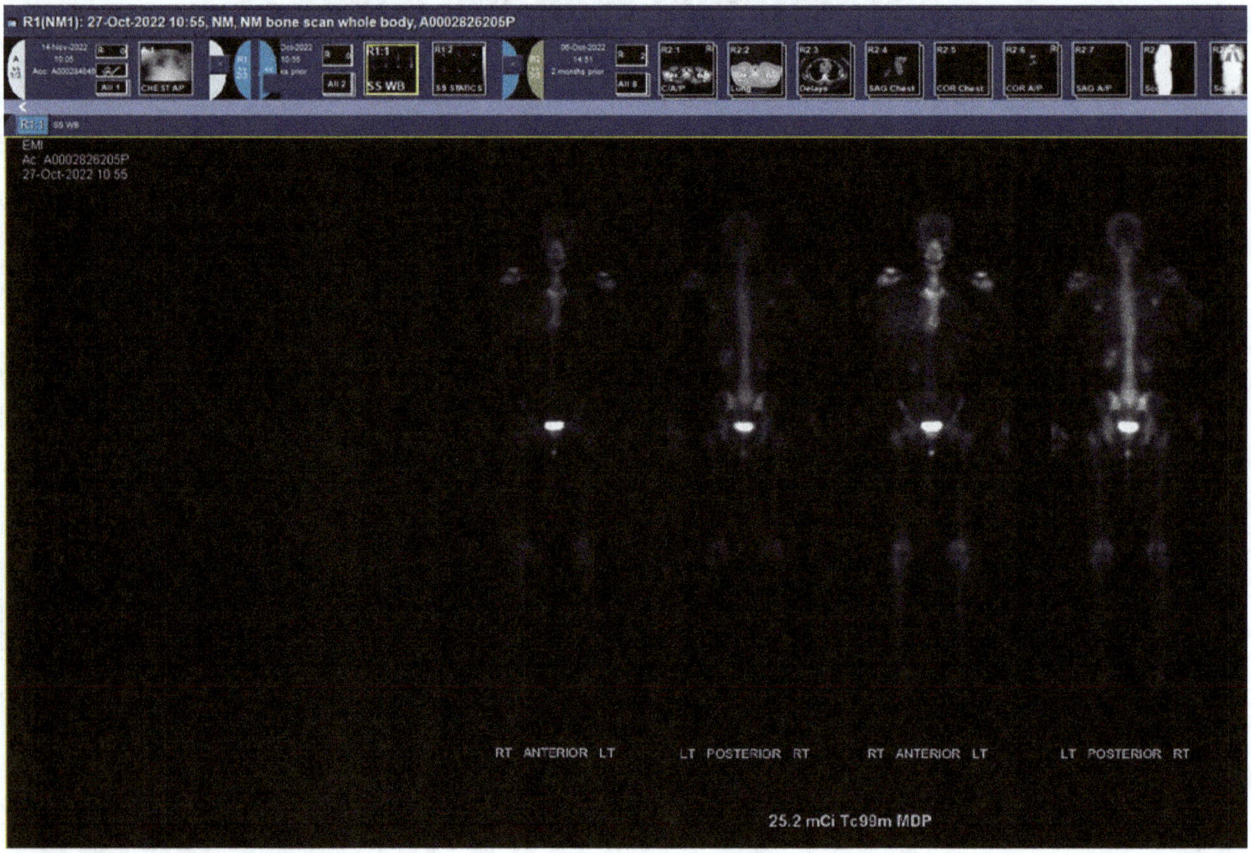

Figure 22.1a CT Scan With IV Contrast

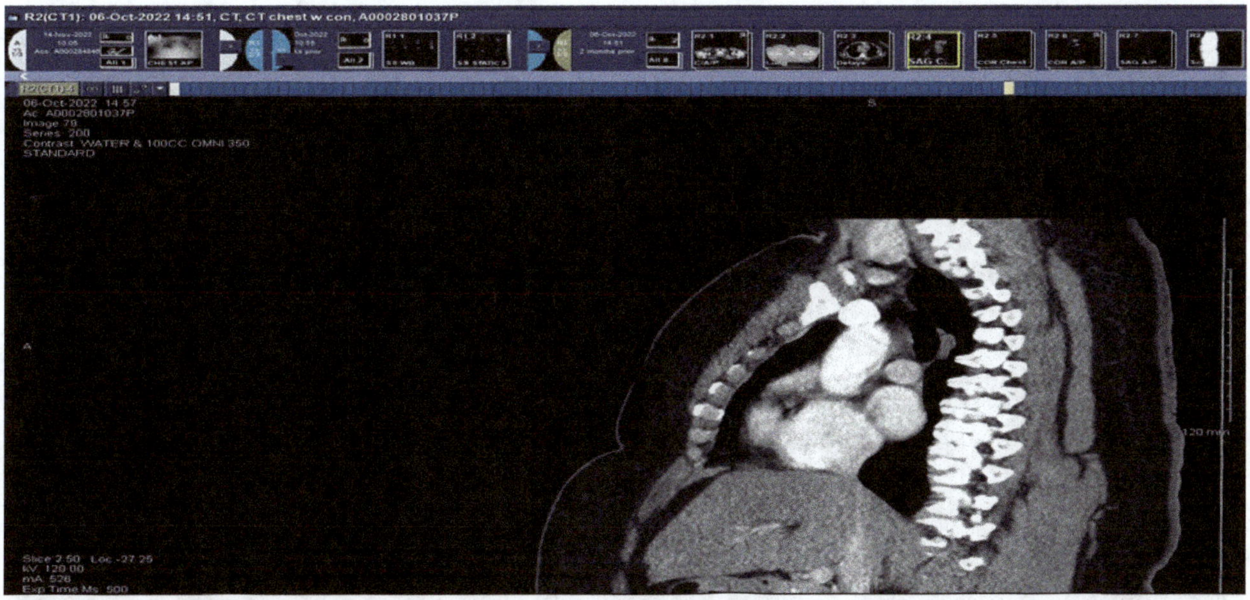

Figure 22.1b CT Scan With IV Contrast

Based on the CT scans, some gastrointestinal abnormalities include hepatomegaly (enlarged liver) and hepatic steatosis (fatty liver disease), and minimal diverticulitis (inflammation in the colon). The patient experienced bone pain, and the bone scans showed a moderate degenerative disc disease with irregular superior endplate and sclerosis.

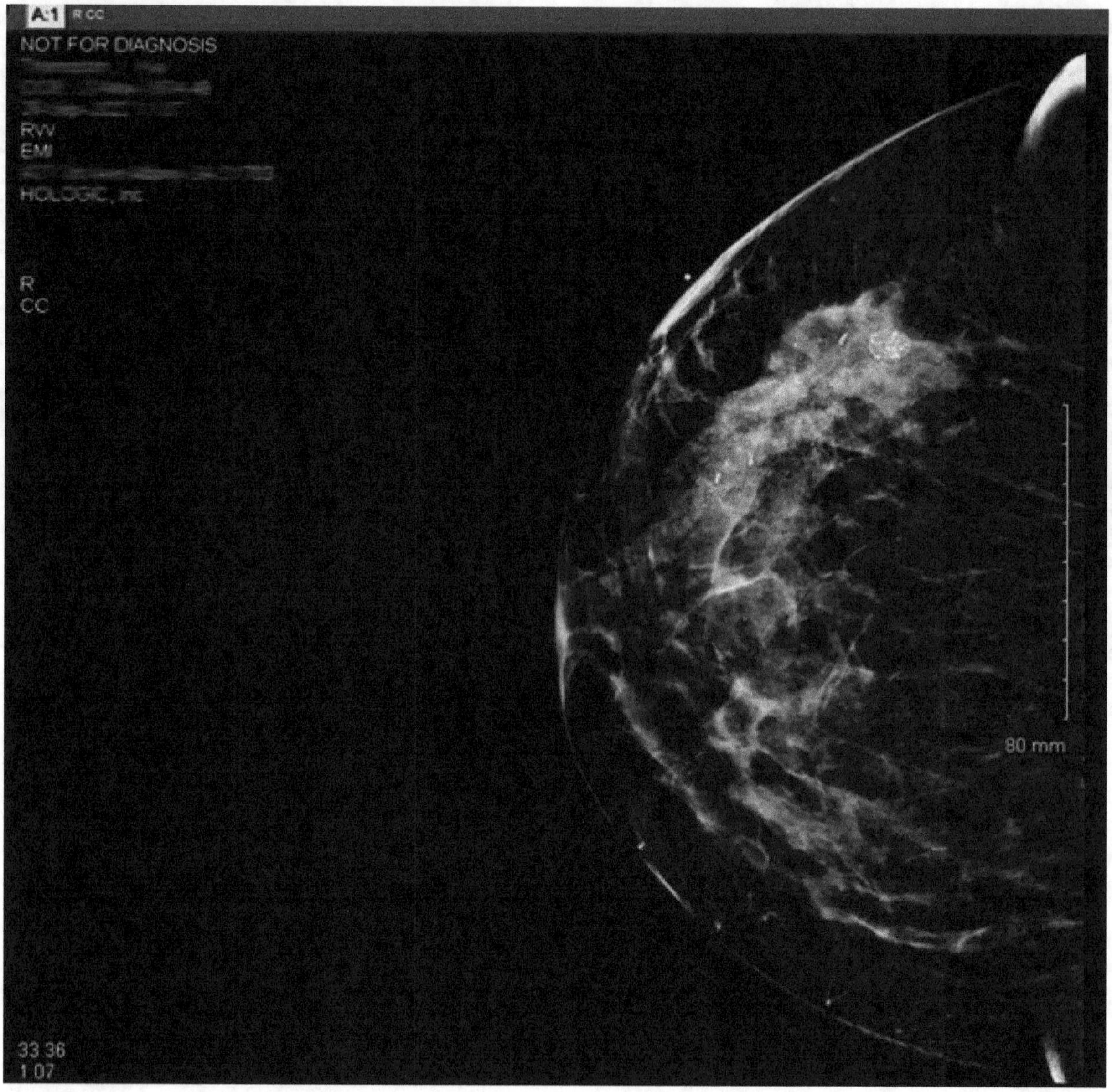

Figure 22.2a

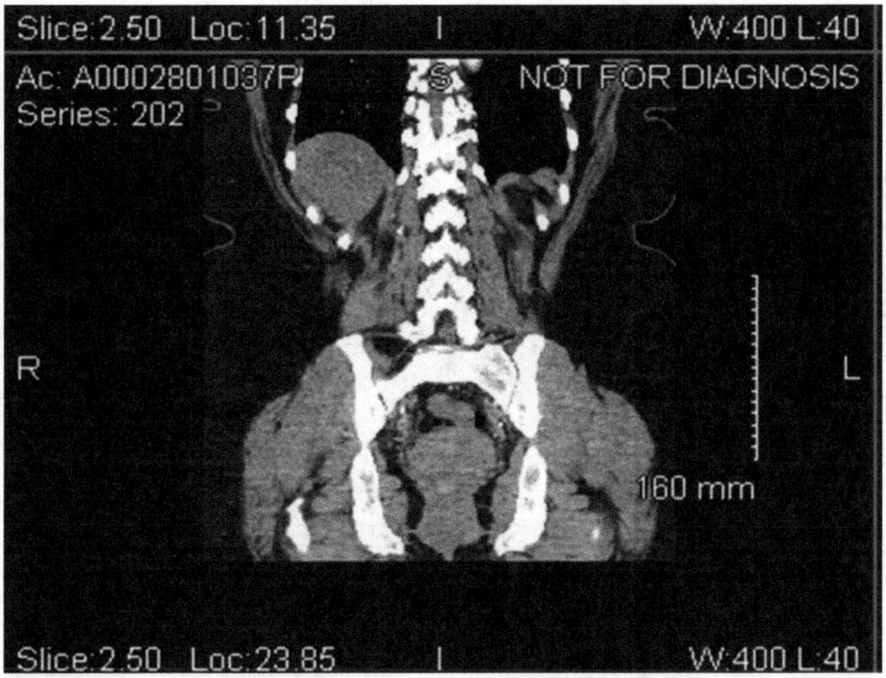

Figure 22.2b

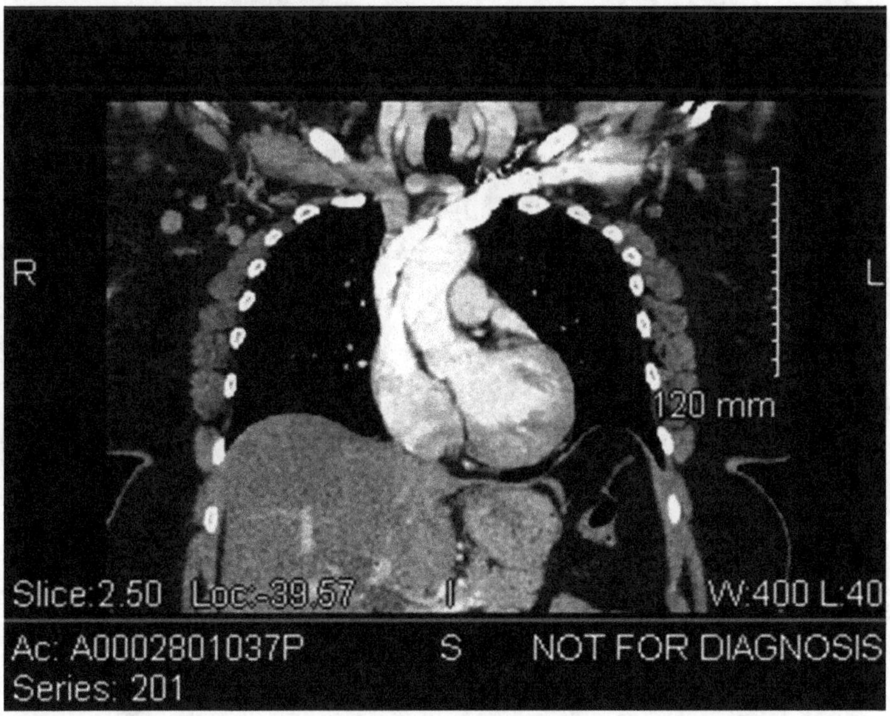

Figure 22.2c

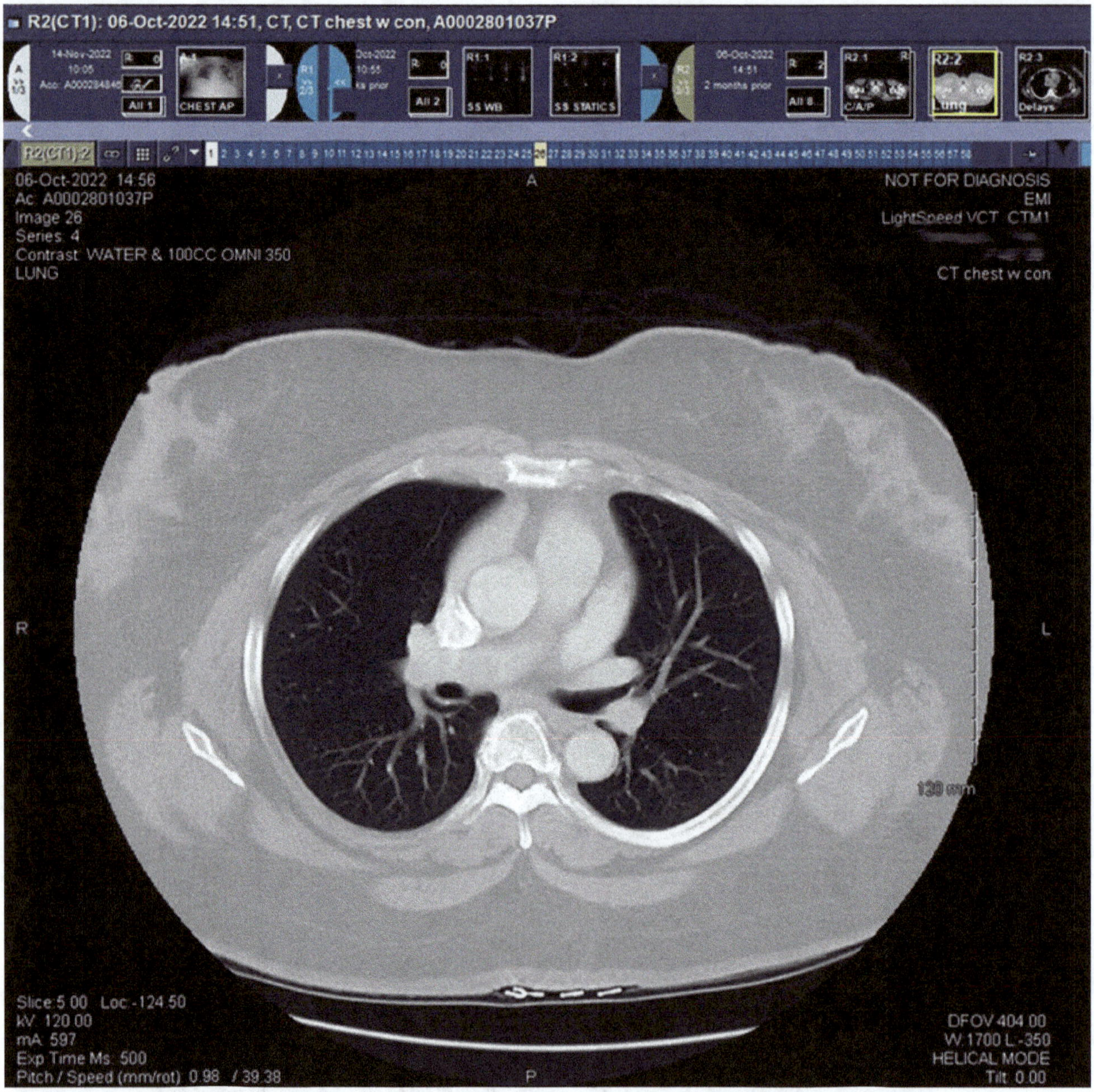

Figure 22.2d CT Scan With IV Contrast

Diagnosis

The patient's breast tissue was biopsied to confirm the presence of cancerous cells in breast lumps.

Estrogen receptor (ER) positive and progesterone receptor (PR) positive. The cancer is responsive to hormone treatment and the prognosis is better than those with ER-negative, PR-negative cancers. HER2 negative means the cancer cells do not have human epidermal growth factor receptor 2. Thus, the cancer is less aggressive than the cancer cells that are HER2-positive. The prognosis is better as well.

Treatment

Breast cancer treatment often consists of surgery to remove the tumor tissue and prevent cancer from spreading. This is done through one of two procedures: a lumpectomy or a mastectomy. A lumpectomy is a breast-conserving surgery that targets the excision to a portion of breast tissue where the lump is located. A mastectomy is the complete surgical removal of one or both breasts and some neighboring lymph nodes. Because of the greater amount of tissue removed around the cancerous cells, a mastectomy is used for high-grade breast cancer cases, as it would reduce the likelihood of recurrence compared to a lumpectomy. On August 28th, 2024, a few lymph nodes were removed. This patient underwent a mastectomy of the right breast to remove cancerous tissue and was followed up with radiation and chemotherapy to ensure cancerous tissue does not return. Chemotherapy medication is used to target and kill cancer cells. For this case a lifeport was implanted in the upper chest to deliver drugs directly into the bloodstream. The function of a lifeport is to maintain vein access during treatment to prevent repeated needle sticks while administering treatment. Alongside the chemotherapy, the patient was also placed on radiation treatment that lasted for 32 rounds from 4/11/23–5/19/24. Radiation therapy works using a beam of high-energy X-rays to destroy cancer cells.

Due to the timely diagnosis and treatment of the cancer, the patient is now in full remission as of August 30, 2024. The mammograms, tests, and scans taken on that day contained no malignancies, as shown in this picture. As for future workup and surveillance, the patient will receive yearly breast mammograms as well as routine annual primary care visits with a blood test.

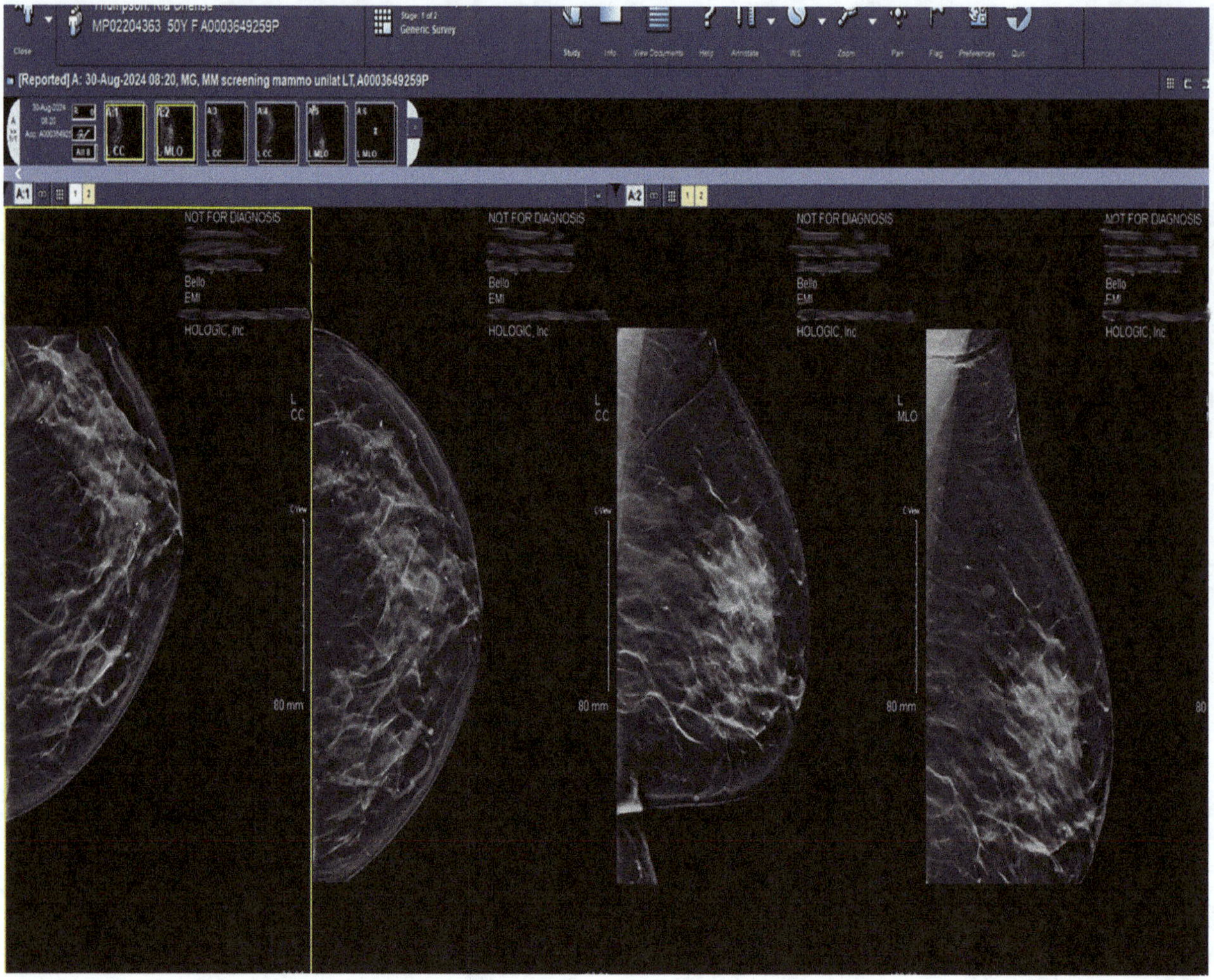

Figure 22.3a Breast CT With Contrast

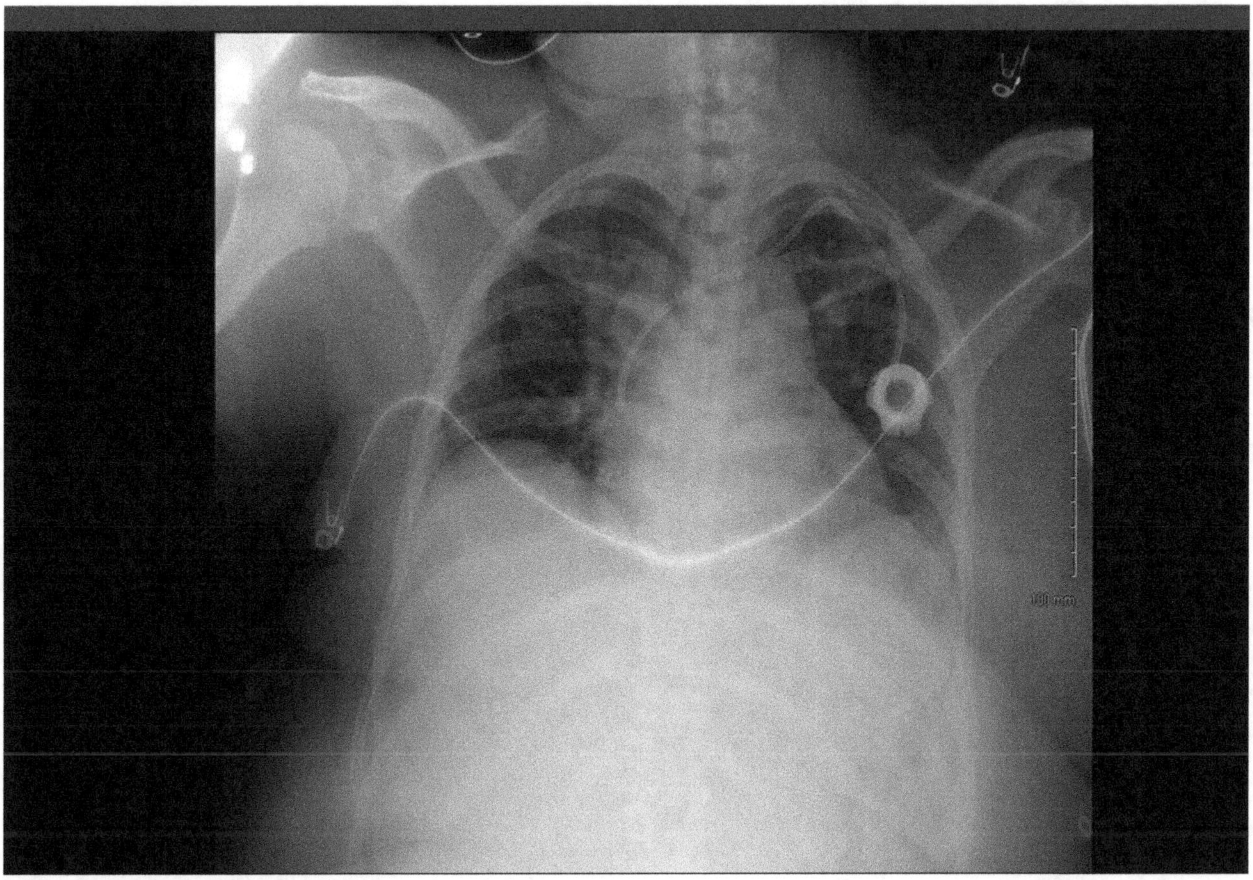

Figure 22.3b Lifeport

What Have We Learned from This Case?

What is breast cancer? Breast cancer is a type of tumor that forms in the cells of the breast. There are different types of tumors such as ductal carcinoma, which starts in ductal epithelial cells, and those that spread to surrounding tissue via metastasis. Secondary tumors caused by metastasis are found in the bone, brain, lung, and liver. Most tumors are unilateral, and incidence increases after age 20. In women, most cases occur between the ages of 50 and 69. In men, cases are less common and found after age 50 as well. Some of the predisposing factors include genetic mutations with BRCA1 and BRCA2, smoking, radiation therapy to the chest, high exposure to estrogen, and close relatives with the disease. Some signs and symptoms include changes on a mammogram or a small, hard, painless nodule. A later sign could be distortion of the breast tissue, dimpled skin, or discharge from the nipple. A biopsy can confirm the presence of cancerous cells. Early detection through regular screenings starting at age 40 can significantly improve the chances of successful treatment and survival rates. Cancer staging is a crucial way to describe the extent of cancer in the body and is important for determining treatment options and prognosis. The system used for staging is the **T**umor, **N**ode, **M**etastasis system. In this system, the tumor part assesses the size and how deeply it has invaded other tissues. The node part evaluates whether the cancer has spread to nearby lymph nodes and the metastasis part indicates whether it has spread to distant parts of the body. The combination of these factors gives us stages from 0 to 5. Stage 0 is localized and noninvasive and stage 5 indicates advanced cancer that has spread to multiple regions of the body.

Other quick facts to note about breast cancer include but are not limited to the following:

- Breast cancer is the most common cancer type in women and accounts for roughly 33% of all new cancer diagnoses in women.
- It also happens to be the deadliest cancer for women if not caught early enough.
- The median age for a diagnosis is 62 years old.
- White women are most at risk for breast cancer.
- Black women typically experience symptoms more severely and have higher morbidity rates for the disease.
- Those who have given birth and breast fed are less at risk of developing the disease.
- Those with immediate family members with the disease are more at risk for developing breast cancer.
- Men can also get diagnosed with breast cancer.

Image Credits

Fig. 22.1a: Copyright © by EMI Group Ltd.

Fig. 22.1b Copyright © by EMI Group Ltd.

Fig. 22.2d: Copyright © by EMI Group Ltd.

Fig. 22.3a: Copyright © by EMI Group Ltd.

Chapter 23

Circulatory System: Case 2

Onset	When the patient was hospitalized for mononucleosis at the age of 16, she was informed that she has biomarkers aligning with hemochromatosis.
Location	
Duration	Has been ongoing since the age of 16 and the patient is 21 years old now.
Characteristic	
Alleviating Factors	Blood donation; herbal remedies to decrease the elevated liver enzymes such as milk thistle, TUDCA, and dandelion root.
Aggravating Factors	Alcohol consumption, excessive dietary intake
Timing	
Severity	

The patient is a 21-year-old Caucasian girl. Some of the patient's family members have hemochromatosis.

Excess iron is usually stored in the skin, heart, liver, pancreas, and joints. Over time, as the liver cannot keep up with the rate of iron deposition, the pancreas begins to start overworking. Elevated pancreatic enzymes usually only occur in patients who have already developed cirrhosis. These complications can be tested with elevated bilirubin, transaminase, amylase, and lipase. Arthritis typically develops 3 to 6 weeks after the peak of the pancreatitis episode and may involve rapid progression to joint damage and pathologic fractures.

Physical Examination

Fatigue, weight loss, weakness, and joint pain, specifically in the fingers.

Diagnosis

Ordered tests include MCH, hemoglobin, red blood cell count, and iron level measurements.

HFE test: a genetic test that looks for mutations in the HFE gene, which encodes the human hemochromatosis protein. The most common mutations are the C282Y and H63D variants.

- In the United States, hereditary hemochromatosis affects 1 in 200–500 people; Most common in people of Northern European descent
- The frequency of the C282Y mutation is 5.4% and the H63D is 13.5%

Treatment

- Giving blood regularly
- Monitoring iron levels
- Dietary considerations
- Monitor liver function

What We Learned

Hemochromatosis is chronic and lifelong once diagnosed. It usually requires ongoing management to prevent iron overload, which leads to a plethora of issues such as diabetes, liver damage, and/or heart failure.

Chapter 24

Musculoskeletal System: Case 3

Onset	A 42-year-old female patient (DOB: 12/15/1981) presents with left TMJ pain for almost 2 years prior to 12/11/2023.
Location	Left masseter, medial pterygoid, and left occipitalis
Duration	The patient has been experiencing pain on the left side of jaw for the last 2 years.
Characteristic	• Chronic pain, which is severe with opening and clenching/closing. • Headaches are located to the left side of her head and left posterior skull and neck. • Pain lasts for >5 hours/day, worsens at night, and radiates to the left occipital and left temporals. • Patient has limited range of motion of the TMJ.
Alleviating Factors	Pain is minimally alleviated with use of NSAIDs.
Aggravating Factors	Patient reports that pain is severe when clenching or opening the mouth.
Timing	Patient reports that the pain persists at rest and worsens at night.
Severity	5/10 throughout the day and 9/10 at night

Temporomandibular joint (TMJ) is the hinge joint that connects the mandibular bone to the temporal bone of the skull. It is known as one of the more complex joints due to its variation in motion. It allows for opening and closing of the mouth, which is also known as hinge action. It allows for sliding of the jaw forward, backward, and side-to-side which is also known as gliding action. Both are important for daily functions such as mastication and speech.

The patient is a nurse who works from home. She reports her job causes stress and makes the pain worse due to her jaw clenching. Patient currently has limited opening and has had limited opening since February 2022. She denies previous history of click or pop of TMJ. However, she had been having left TMJ pain for 6–12 months prior to February 2022. Patient reports clenching throughout the day. She previously had an occlusal appliance for more than 3 years and reports minimal benefit and poor fit. NSAIDs provide minimal benefits, and she has not tried muscle relaxants. Patient states that she has a limited range of motion in her jaw that has caused her trouble with eating.

Past Medical History

- HTN, hypothyroidism, GERD, gastric ulcers, recurrent Clostridioides difficile infections (cleared November 7, 2023)
- Denies head and neck trauma
- Denies a history of open lock
- Surgeries: Tonsillectomy, adenoidectomy (2011), hysterectomy and oophorectomy (2013), rotator cuff surgery (2019)

Medications: Adderall XR, Lasix, Nebivolol, Syntrhoid, Topamax, Vitamin D3, Zoloft

Social History

- Smoking: Denies
- Alcohol: Denies
- Illicit drugs: Denies

Physical Exam and Tests

December 11, 2023

- Pain with palpation of extraoral muscles of mastication: left temporalis, left masseter, left occipitalis, left scalene
- Pain with palpation of intraoral muscles of mastication
- Intraoral: wear facets noted
- Maximal incisal opening (MIO) without pain is 28 mm; no popping or clicking appreciated; deviation to the left on opening
- MIO with pain is 34 mm; no popping or clicking; deviation to the left on opening
- Left lateral excursion: 7 mm with pain
- Right lateral excursion: 8 mm with pain
- Left occlusal loading: left-sided TMJ pain noted along with left masseter pain
- Right occlusal loading: left-sided TMJ pain noted; left masseter pain
- Auscultation: no appreciable crepitus noted

Radiographic: Narrow joint space noted bilaterally; no cortical erosions; no osteolytic or osteoblastic processes noted. Bilaterial maxillary sinuses appear clear.

Impression:

- Acute closed lock versus myofascial pain and muscle spasms
- Patient does have myofascial symptoms

Plan

- Recommend the patient obtain a splint from the dentist
    - Splint to be full coverage, custom, hard, monoplane, flat occlusal surface appliance; worn 24 hours/day for the first month then nightly; increase wear at tiems of increased muscle pain/stress
- Soft diet, warm compresses, stress relieving activity (yoga, swimming, massage, etc.)
- Muscle relaxants
- Will plan for MRI to rule out anterior disc displacement

MRI was done on January 10, 2024: Findings concerning for partial disruption involving the posterior margin of the left TMJ disc.
On January 29, 2024

- Pain with palpation in left masseter, medial pterygoid, left occipitalis
- Pain with palpation of intraoral sites
- Mouth open without pain: 23 mm
- Mouth open with pain: 28 mm with left deviation
- Right lateral excursion of 6 mm
- Left lateral excursion of 10 mm
- Right occlusal loading: left jaw pain

Treatments

Left arthrocentesis was done on 2/20/2024 with manipulation of the TMJ followed by possible physical therapy.

Flexeril (muscle relaxer)

Patient still reports severe pain in the left TMJ; pain persists at night; muscle relaxers have offered no relief.

TMJ disorders affect the normal range of motion of the joint and can cause pain in the jaw and surrounding structures.

Signs and symptoms of TMJ syndrome include the following:

- Pain or tenderness in the jaw
- Pain in both or one temporomandibular joint
- Aching in or around ears
- Facial pain
- Locked joint making it difficult to open or close the mouth

What Have We Learned from this Case?

Temporomandibular joint syndrome, also known as TMJ syndrome or temporomandibular joint disorder (abbreviated TMD).

- TMJ syndrome is a disorder of the temporomandibular joint.
- TMJ syndrome limits the normal range of motion and causes pain as well as inflammation of the surrounding tissues and muscles.
- It can occur from damage to the articular disc, which acts as a shock absorber for jaw movements, erosion of the cartilage or bone, overuse of muscles associated with mastication like the masseter muscle, and bruxism or grinding of the teeth.

- The specific cause of TMJ syndrome is often difficult to determine with the many factors at play. Some factors are mechanical stress like jaw clenching, trauma to the jaw from falls or injury, malocclusion of the teeth, and degenerative diseases like rheumatoid arthritis. Psychological factors can also contribute to the development of TMJ syndrome such as stress can lead to muscle tension and clenching.
- The symptoms of TMJ syndrome are localized pain or tenderness in the jaw, aching pain around the face especially around the ears, difficulty chewing, difficulty opening and closing mouth, jaw locking, and clicking or popping sounds during jaw movement.

TMJ can be diagnosed by a TMJ specialist or dentist through various physical and imaging tests.

- The physical tests that can be done are palpation of the face and jaw in which areas of tenderness, tightness, and pain are assessed. The range of motion test is done to observe the extent the patient can move and open and close their jaw to assess any tightness or pain.
- Imaging techniques used to diagnose TMJ include dental X-rays to examine teeth and jaw, CT scan to provide images of bones, MRI to detect inflammation and swelling, and arthroscopy, which is a tube put into an incision in the jaw through mouth to take images of the damage at the joint.

Treatments for TMJ include medications and physical remedies.

- Medications one can take for TMJ are pain relievers such as NSAIDs and acetaminophen. Muscle relaxers can be taken to relax jaw muscles and alleviate pain. Botox would relax the muscles around the jaw to prevent nerve signals that cause painful contractions.
- Physical remedies include wearing a mouth guard to sleep to realign the jaw joint and reduce pressure, which would help alleviate pain, and physical therapy to strengthen the jaw and improve function.
- Arthrocentesis would wash out any inflammatory or harmful materials in the jaw joint by injecting sterile saline.

Chapter 25

Musculoskeletal System: Case 4

Onset	A small lump was formed when the patient was 6 years old and had grown to the size of a golf ball causing discomfort with shoes.
Location	Under left ankle
Duration	Has been with the lump since he was 6 years old, and he is 21 years old now.
Characteristic	The lump causes a moderate discomfort only during exercise. Discomfort and dull pain normally only lasts a few minutes. The mass is a hard, solid lump.
Alleviating Factors	Ibuprofen or other pain medication
Aggravating Factors	Exercise
Timing	The pain is intermittent but would occur with engaging activities such as playing soccer. There is little to no pain with normal daily activities.
Severity	

Physical Examination

The left ankle function remains intact. The lump was solid and measured to be roughly the size of a golf ball. The patient reports little to no pain when the lump is touched.

Diagnostic Tests

MRI shows that the lump is localized to the ankle and appears to affect peroneal tendons. It was found to be directly on top of the tendons but not connected to them.

Then the patient was referred to an orthopedic surgeon at Children's Hospital of Atlanta. A tumor excision and biopsy were done.

There are two peroneal tendons: the peroneus brevis and longus. The peroneal tendons are located in the lower leg, run down the outside of the ankle, and attach to the foot. They stabilize the ankle and help pull the foot outward and downward.

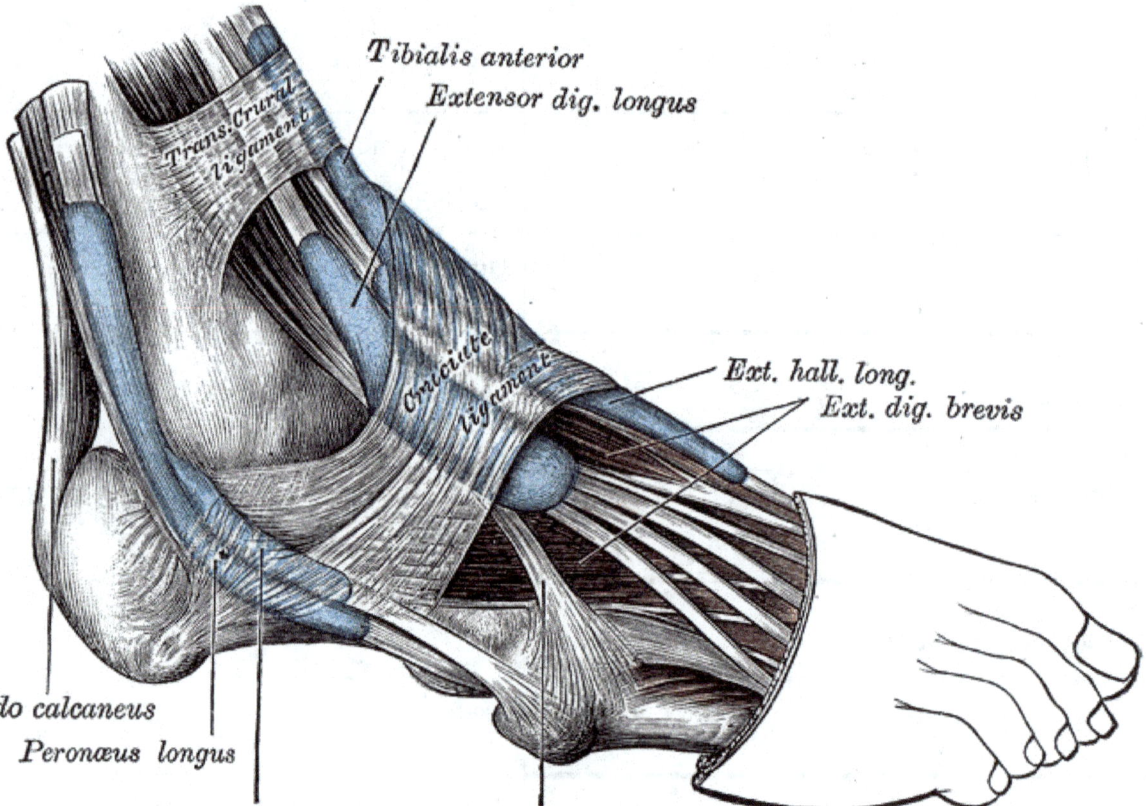

Figure 25.1 Peroneal Tendons 1

Treatment

Initial excision and biopsy appeared to be normal. Six weeks later, the pathologist went back and reexamined the mass, and a diagnosis of clear cell sarcoma (CCS) was made. The patient was brought back for tumor bed resection. Peroneal tendons were included, so corresponding reconstruction was done. The patient also underwent two lymphadenectomies following suspicious PET scans, which proved to be benign.

- CCS is rare soft tissue cancer that grows just below the skin
- CCS occurs most often in the arms, legs, feet, and hands
- CCS can grow throughout the torso, specifically to the stomach and intestines, and also to the head and genitalia
- It is an exceedingly aggressive tumor, accounting for 1% of soft tissue sarcomas
- There is a 5-year survival rate of 50%–69%

- CCS is common in younger adults, typically being found in adults in their 20s to 40s
- It is treated with surgery as radiation & chemo therapies are not very effective against CCS. The best way to treat CCS is to remove the entire tumor.
- CCS has very few signs or symptoms. It appears as a small nodule and does not cause any significant symptoms until it has spread, or rather metastasized, to other areas of the body

The patient was monitored with PET scans every 3 months for a year to monitor possible spread of malignancy. The patient also did blood tests to monitor the malignancy. MRI and CT of foot and chest were performed every 6 months. The patient was deemed cancer free at the age of 18.

The patient was prescribed an antidepressant and insomnia medication during cancer treatment. Amitriptyline is prescribed at 50 milligrams. The patient was also told to get yearly imaging done of the original tumor site and chest to ensure the tumor does not recur.

Image Credits

Fig. 25.1: Henry Vandyke Carter, https://commons.wikimedia.org/wiki/File:Gray441.png, 1918.

Chapter 26

Nervous System: Case 3

Onset	A newborn has muscle weakness, vision problems, and cognitive difficulties
Location	
Duration	Seizures are still ongoing since she was born.
Characteristic	Sharp and throbbing pain due to muscle weakness when attending physical therapy.
Alleviating Factors	Clobazam helps control seizures and muscle spasms. Specific positioning and still movements can help alleviate the pain.
Aggravating Factors	Loud noise and laying on her back for long period of time. Physical activity involving stretching can cause more pain.
Timing	The pain is intermittent when seizures occur.
Severity	The pain ranges from mild to severe.

She was born with hydrocephalus and was not expected to live more than 24 hours. She is now 5 years old.

Hydrocephalus is characterized by the abnormal buildup of cerebrospinal fluid (CSF) in the brain's ventricles. The extra fluid puts pressure on the brain and can cause brain damage. It is also characterized by head enlargement in infants. The two images show how the brain of a baby with hydrocephalus might look compared to a brain without.

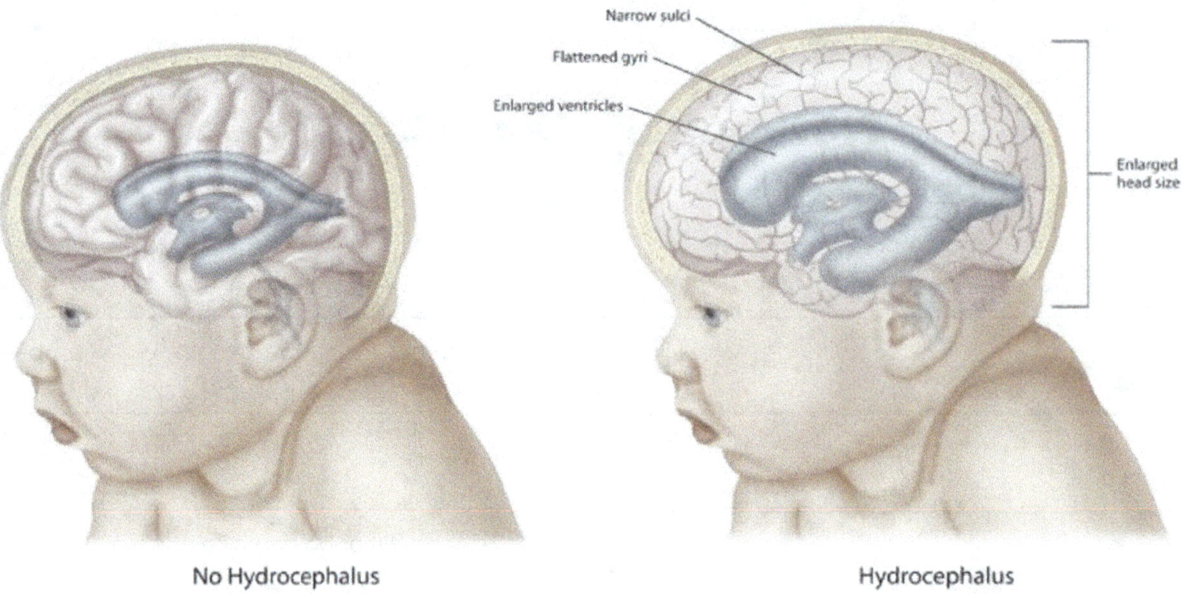

Figure 26.1 Normal Versus Brain with Hydrocephalus 1

At 1 day old, the head ultrasound) was normal. A head ultrasound (HUS) is a diagnostic tool used to detect intraventricular hemorrhage (IVH) in babies. At 2 days old, the HUS showed a grade 2 IVH. This indicates bleeding inside the ventricles, but there is no ventricular dilatation. The image shows what a grade 2 IVH would look like compared to a normal scan. 1 week old, the HUS showed bilateral grade 3 IVH and decreased pulsation. This indicates bleeding enlarging the ventricles by more than 50%. At 2 weeks old, an MRI marked expansion of all lateral ventricles with blood and CSF with marked hydrocephalus. This means the ventricles have become significantly larger than normal with bleeding in the brain and confirms hydrocephalus diagnosis. At 3 weeks old, a fast sequence MRI showed continued enlarged ventricles. A subgaleal shunt was placed. Around 6 weeks old, the head circumference was measured at 35 cm. A fast sequence MRI showed improved ventriculomegaly and improved mass effect over the brainstem. This indicates the shunt is working. For the future: fast sequence MRI is recommended to visualize CSF spaces and monitor hydrocephalus. A CT scan is recommended to monitor structural brain changes to assess whether the hydrocephalus is obstructive. Single-photon emission CT (SPECT) and PET scans can evaluate brain metabolism or blood flow. Visual evoked potential (VEP) and somatosensory evoked potential (SSEP) can assess how well the brain is responding to sensory input.

On April 7, 2019, the patient was born via C-section due to placental abruption and non-reassuring fetal heart rate tracing (NRFHT). NRFHT refers to an abnormal fetal heart rate pattern observed during labor or delivery that may indicate a potential problem with the baby's oxygen supply. The patient had APGAR Scores of 0, 2, 3, 4. The APGAR scores assess the newborn's health (on a scale from 1 to 10). The patient experienced dangerously low scores, indicating a need for immediate medical attention. On April 15, 2019, an echocardiogram showed mild right ventricular hypertrophy and septal hypertrophy. A repeat echocardiogram was normal. On May 15, 2019, a hearing screen showed no concerns. On May 22, 2019, a slow-flow heart murmur was detected. It is recommended to check for abnormal heart rate, respiratory rate, or oxygen saturation. Continual ECG is also recommended if the murmur worsens.

The patient was intubated at birth on April 7, 2019. On April 8, 2019, the patient was extubated to noninvasive mechanical ventilation (NIMV). On April 15, 2019, nasal continuous positive airway pressure (NCPAP) supported with high-flow nasal cannula (HFNC) was used to maintain stable blood gases. NCPAP maintains a constant pressure in the patient's airways, helping to keep the alveoli open. HFNC delivers a high flow of oxygen to the patient through a nasal cannula and provides both humidification and positive pressure. Stable blood gases mean the patient's oxygen, carbon dioxide, pH, and bicarbonate levels are within an acceptable range, and there are no immediate concerns for respiratory acidosis or alkalosis. The acceptable/normal ranges for infants are as follows:

- pH range: 7.35–7.45
- PaCO2 (carbon dioxide): 35–45 mmHg
- PaO2 (oxygen): 50–70 mmHg (term infant)
- HCO3 (bicarbonate): 22–26 mEq/L
- Oxygen saturation (SaO2): 92%–94%

On April 26, 2019, flow weaned to 1, indicating recovery. On April 27, 2019, the patient put on room air with stable follow-up gases. The patient's respiratory distress was resolved.

Nutrition

Nil per os (NPO) means nothing by mouth at birth. The patient received total parenteral nutrition (TPN) from April 8, 2019, to April 21, 2019. On April 25, 2019, feeds were changed to EnfaCare 24 cal/oz on admission to the children's hospital in Atlanta. Poly-vi-sol was started, which is a liquid multivitamin supplement. On May 4, 2019, feeds were changed to continuous due to emesis. On May 6, 2019, occupational therapy was consulted for oral skills. On May 7, 2019, a transpyloric tube was placed under fluoroscopy due to continued emesis. On May 9, 2019, a swallow study is unable to be completed due to numerous gagging episodes without any sucking attempt elicited. On May 14, 2019, a fundoplication and gastrostomy tube was placed.

Seizures

On April 11, 2019, moderate to severe diffuse cortical dysfunction and irritability, clinical seizures with and without EEG correlates.

On April 17, 2019, moderate diffuse cortical dysfunction and irritability, episodes of focal, and right hemispheric electrographic seizures.

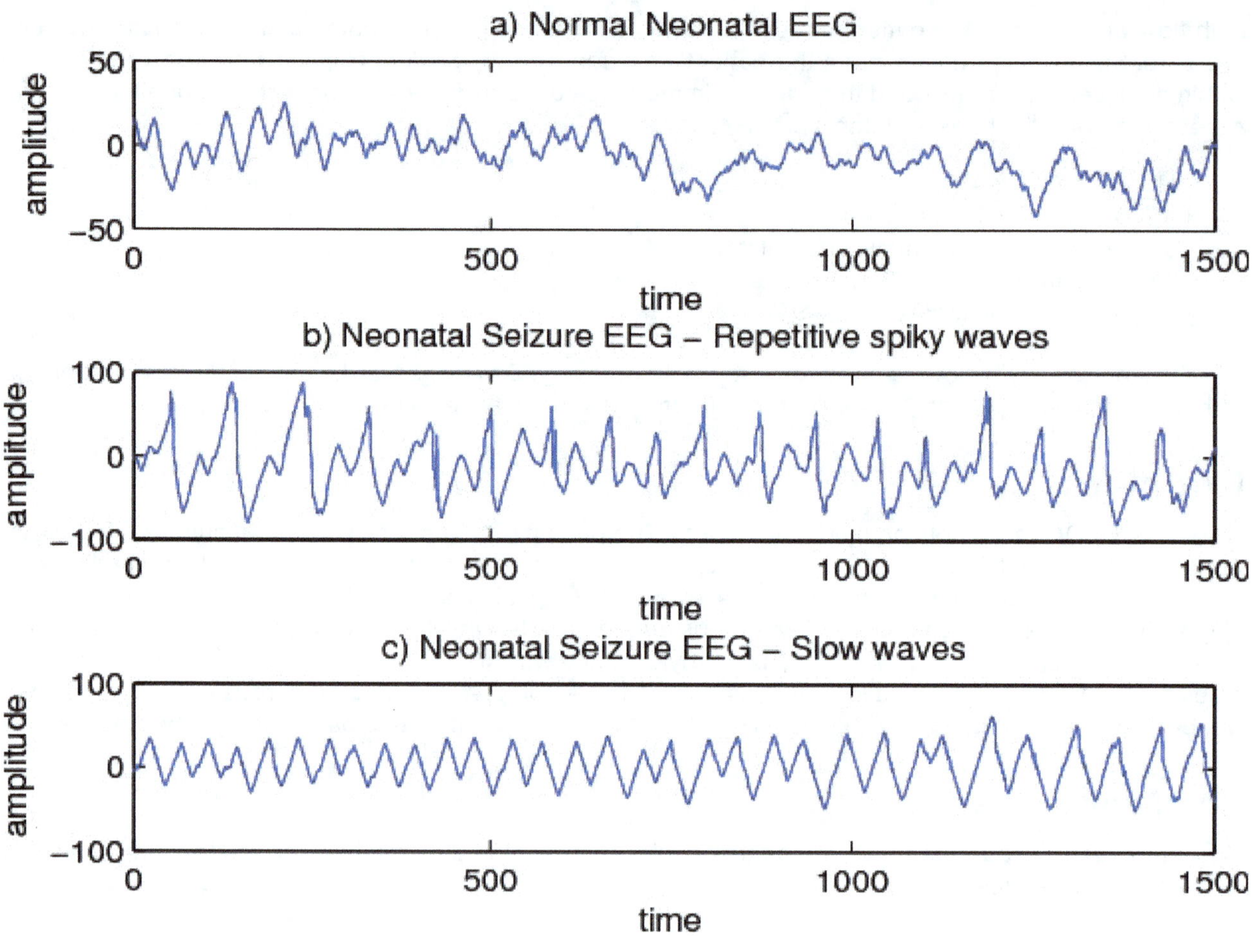

Figure 26.2 Normal and Neonatal Seizure EEG

Adrenal Hemorrhage

On April 26, 2019, abdominal ultrasound showed septated cystic mass in the right upper quadrant. The mass showed no internal blood flow, indicating a likely adrenal hemorrhage. A CT scan was ordered and a mass observed (like a hemorrhage)

On May 2, 2019, renal ultrasound showed a likely resolving hematoma that appeared smaller than on the previous ultrasound.

On May 21, 2019, renal ultrasound showed interval decrease in the size of the heterogeneous right suprarenal lesion which may represent adrenal hemorrhage.

Treatment

For treatment of hydrocephalus, excess CSF was drained through several shunt placements. Initially, a bilateral subgaleal shunt was placed as a safer temporary measure on April 30, 2019, considering the patient's age and incidence of an intraventricular hemorrhage. On May 14, 2019, a fundoplication was performed to prevent gastric reflux, and a gastrostomy tube was placed for feeds. On July 2, 2019, the temporary shunt was removed and subsequently replaced with a more permanent shunt option to drain CSF, known as a ventriculoperitoneal (VP) shunt. The shunt must be maintained and ventricular pressure monitored to ensure the safety of the patient. (On August 7, 2019, a VP shunt exploration and revision was done.) An external ventricular drainage (EVD) was also placed and eventually removed. On August 20, 2019, an EVD was removed, and right VP shunt was placed. An EVD is an external, temporary shunt where CSF is drained externally, so pressure, the amount of CSF drained, and the contents of the CSF can be routinely evaluated.

Other Surgeries

- On August 11, 2020, supraglottoplasty was done.
- On May 26, 2022, a right inguinal hernia was repaired.
- On October 10, 2023, left pelvic and proximal femoral osteotomy, left adductor release, bilateral hamstring lengthening, and bilateral percutaneous Achilles lengthening were done.

All of the following have been and will continue to be provided to improve the patient's quality of life and treat outcomes of the patient's cerebral palsy.

Current medication: Famotidine (for acid reflux), Keppra (for seizures), Clobazam (for muscle spasms and seizure control), Glycopyrrolate (to reduce saliva and drooling), and Gabapentin (to treat epilepsy)

Regular monitoring of the child's growth and nutrition needs, with possible changes in the feeding tube formula or feeding schedule. Introduction of oral feeding trials if the child can tolerate it, with help from therapists and dietitians.

Ongoing physical therapy to help with muscle stiffness and improve movement, focusing on stretching and keeping muscles flexible. Occupational therapy to improve feeding skills and fine motor skills, especially because of the child's challenges with oral feeding and the need for a feeding tube.

Possible future VP shunt adjustments or replacements as the child grows, especially if there are issues with the shunt's function or infection. Potential orthopedic surgeries to help with tight muscles or joint problems caused by cerebral palsy, like tendon releases or bone surgeries. Regular MRI or CT scans to check the shunt, manage hydrocephalus, and monitor any brain changes. Follow-up abdominal scans to make sure the adrenal hemorrhage is healing and to check for any new concerns. EEG tests to track seizure activity and brain function, especially if there are changes in how often seizures happen.

Image Credits

Fig. 26.1: Centers for Disease Control and Prevention, National Center on Birth Defects and Developmental Disabilities, https://commons.wikimedia.org/wiki/File:Hydrocephalus_CDC.png, U.S. Department of Health and Human Services, 2013.

Fig. 26.2: Kok-Kiong Poh and Pina Marziliano, "Analysis of Neonatal EEG Signals using Stockwell Transform," Annual International Conference of the IEEE Engineering in Medicine and Biology Society. Copyright © 2007 by Inscribe Publications.

Chapter 27

HEENT: Case 2

Onset	The patient had blurry vision/vision loss in the upper 2 quadrants of the right eye for over 3 days. Ocular discomfort as well as retro-orbital pain were felt with ocular movements and right sided facial movements.
Location	Upper 2 quadrants of the right eye
Duration	8 days
Characteristics	Top half of the right eye vision field is completely gone; Blurred vision worsens over time with increasing vision loss; no pain
Alleviating/Aggravating Factors	None
Timing	NA
Severity	Moderate

The patient is a 21-year-old White female who presented to the emergency room with an elevated blood pressure and right eye blurriness/vision loss in the upper quadrants for over 3 days. She woke up with blurry vision in her right eye, and while at work she tried to flush the eye with normal saline to help and did not work. 2 days later she went to see the optometrist who then noticed she had elevated blood pressure and recommended that she go to the emergency room due to a concern for ischemic retinopathy or other acute processes.

Medical History: she does not wear glasses or has any vision difficulty. The patient had general anxiety disorder but not hypertension.

Family History: Her parents do not wear glasses; however, diabetes, hyperlipidemia, and hypertension run in her family.

Physical Examination:

Elevated blood pressure and heart rate

Differential blood count: low lymphocyte/high neutrophil

Hematology: High sedimentation rate, low albumin, low Hgb

Special chemistry: High C reactive protein

Lipids: High cholesterol

Anti-nuclear Ab: negative

Treponema pallidum Ab: non-reactive

Head CT: unremarkable

MRI with contrast: unremarkable

Echocardiogram: unremarkable

Agitated saline contrast echocardiography: unremarkable

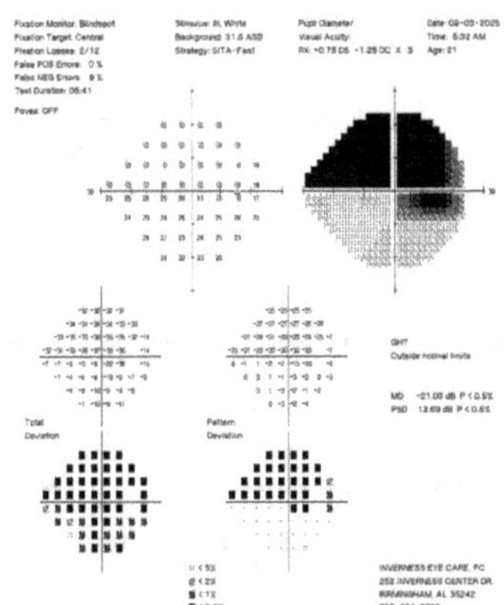

Figure 27.1 Black areas represent vision loss or blurry vision.

Treatment:

Surgery: not required

The first step of treatment is using steroids to treat inflammation. Next step is inpatient, followed by outpatient, hyperbaric chamber sessions to help restore oxygen flow to the patient's eye. Before discharge, the patient continued to receive IV Solu-Medrol, which is an IV steroid used to treat inflammatory and autoimmune conditions. Additionally, the patient started taking aspirin for ischemic prophylaxis and was advised to avoid taking estrogen-containing oral contraceptive pills, which may have contributed to this ischemic event. An outpatient transesophageal endoscopy was scheduled to see if the patient has a patent foramen ovale that might be the case of the blockage of oxygen.

For the hyperbaric chamber sessions, the oxygen level was 3 atmospheric pressures. 5-minute breaks with normal oxygen pressure were taken every 30 minutes. After completing 9 successful hyperbaric

chamber sessions, the patient experienced an absent seizure. Then the scheduled 10th hyperbaric chamber session was cancelled.
Medications: ferrous sulfate, prednisone, pantoprazole

Zoloft: 100 mg for anxiety
The patient had 95% of her vision restored after the chamber treatments. However, her optic nerve suffered some damage. Systemic risk factors should be well controlled for a stable prognosis.
Ischemic optic neuropathy (ION) is a condition which results from inadequate blood supply to the optic nerve, causing sudden vision loss. The optic nerve requires an ample blood supply for its function. When the blood flow is blocked, optic nerve fibers become ischemic and then the function is impaired. ION can be categorized as either anterior, affecting the optic nerve head, or posterior, affecting optic nerve behind the optic disc. ION can also be categorized to arteritic and non-arteritic. Arteritic ION results from inflammation of an artery near the optic nerve, typically caused by giant cell arteritis. Non-arteritic ION is linked to systemic vascular risk (for example, atherosclerosis, diabetes, embolization, or trauma).
Risk factors for ION include

- systemic hypertension, diabetes mellitus, hyperlipidemia, obstructive sleep apnea, smoking, advanced age
- small, crowded disc anatomy
- autoimmune vasculitis (for instance, giant cell arteritis)

Symptoms of ION always include vision loss caused by a lack of blood flow to the optic nerve, but some differ depending on which category the ION falls into. Non-arteritic anterior ION, the most common form, causes sudden or rapid onset and painless vision loss, presenting as blurring or worsened vision across part of the field of view. This usually affects one eye at a time, and most people first notice the loss of vision when waking up. Arteritic anterior ION causes sudden vision loss including blurring, darkening or dimming, worsening vision or complete vision loss, often accompanied by headache, malaise, and swollen arteries in the temples. Posterior ION also causes sudden, painless vision loss, but the symptoms get worse in the initial phase.

ION can be diagnosed through ophthalmic and imaging tests as well as lab tests. A fundoscopic exam would show a swollen optic disc with segmental edema and splinter hemorrhages. An optical coherence tomography scan would show acute thickening of the retinal nerve fiber followed by thinning over time due to axonal loss. Visual field testing would show loss of vision in either the upper or lower half of the visual field, and a Fluorescein Angiography would show delayed or incomplete filling of the optic disc circulation. Laboratory tests would be used to determine if the ION is arteritic, where elevated erythrocyte sedimentation rate, C-Reactive Protein and thrombocytosis would provide evidence for systemic inflammation, pointing towards giant cell arteritis. Other tests include intraocular pressure test, Optical Coherence Tomography (OCT) showing thinning of nerve fiber from axonal loss, Visual Field-Testing showing loss in upper or lower half of field, ultrasound and/or MRI of nearby blood vessels to identify blockage.

Lifestyle changes and modifiable factors for prevention of ION include controlling blood pressure, managing diabetes, lowering cholesterol, treating sleep apnea, smoking secession, and exercising regularly. Because vision loss from ION is typically irreversible, education focuses on reducing recurrence and protecting the unaffected eye.

Patients are advised to manage modifiable vascular risk factors. This includes maintaining stable and healthy blood pressure, avoiding excessive drops in nighttime blood pressure, and monitoring readings regularly. For those with diabetes, good glycemic control is essential. The management of high cholesterol through diet, reduced saturated fat intake, and the use of prescribed statins is also important. Sleep apnea is recognized as a major risk factor, so screening and treatment are recommended for affected patients. Smoking cessation is strongly encouraged to improve overall vascular health and reduce optic nerve ischemia.

Additional recommendations include engaging in regular physical activity, following a balanced diet, and attending routine follow-up visits with ophthalmology and primary care. Patients are instructed to seek immediate medical attention if they notice any new or sudden vision changes. Overall, the educational focus is on long-term vascular health and prevention of further ischemic events.

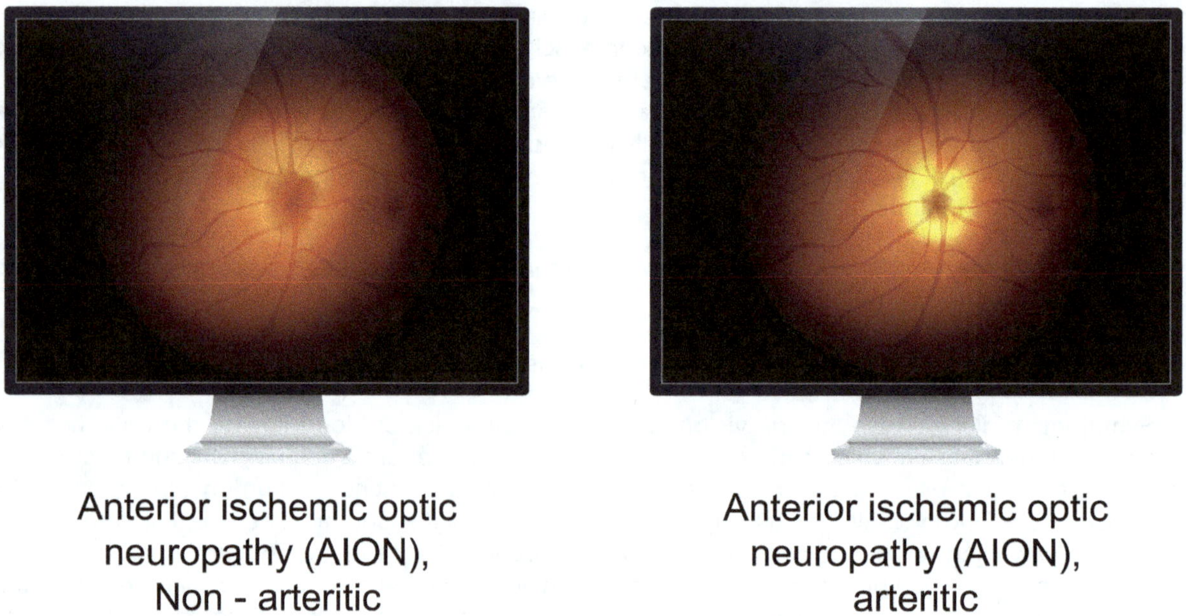

Figure 27.2 Ischemic optic neuropathy

Image Credits

Chapter 28

Musculoskeletal System: Case 5

Onset	General muscle weakness and vision difficulty in his left eye.
Location	Drooping of eyelids.
Duration	2 months.
Characteristics	Fatigue gets progressively worse with repetitive activities, drooping of eyelids, double vision, progressive difficulty with chewing.
Alleviating/aggravating factors	Activities that required sustained muscle use aggravated the weakness, while rest and prescribed medication (pyridostigmine) provided relief.
Timing	Symptoms were most noticeable in the evening after daily activities. Some improvements were seen in the morning.
Severity	Moderate but significantly interfering with daily tasks such as eating and reading.

A 74-year-old White male checked into the emergency room with a chief compliant of general muscle weakness and difficulty seeing with his left eye. The symptoms have been present for 2 months, and his condition has slowly worsened. The patient reported a gradual onset of symptoms over the course of 2 months. Initially, he noticed drooping of the eyelids (ptosis) and double vision. His symptoms would later progress to general muscle weakness, especially in the muscles of the jaw, shoulders, and diaphragm.

The patient felt fatigue, which got worsened throughout the day but better with rest.

The patient has a history of high blood pressure, for which he takes Losartan daily.

Physical Examination:

The patient demonstrated bilateral eyelid drooping (ptosis) that worsened with sustained upward gaze and intermittent diplopia on lateral gaze. Speech was slightly slurred, and he reported fatigue with chewing solid foods. Strength testing was performed, which revealed proximal muscle weakness in the shoulders and hips that worsened after repeated exertion. Sensory examination and deep tendon reflexes were normal.

Lab tests:

CBC with differentials, BMP, TSH/Free T4, AchR antibody tests, EMG

Serum anticholinergic antibody test: Positive

EMG: A decreased neuromuscular response

- The patient had a >15% decrement in compound muscle action potential amplitude.
    - Indicates extensive muscle weakness.
- Of the single fiber EMG, the patient had increased jitter and blocking present.
    - Indicates a decrease in the strength of the electrical signal as it travels along the nerve.

Treatment:

To treat his myasthenia gravis, the patient was prescribed once daily pyridostigmine. This medication is an acetylcholinesterase inhibitor. By inhibiting the breakdown of acetylcholine in the neuromuscular junction, the muscles can be activated even though they have less functional acetylcholine receptors.

Blepharoplasty

Possible differential diagnosis:

ALS, stroke, MS, myasthenia gravis

Prognosis:

- It has now been 12 months since the patient was originally presented to the emergency room.
- He has been taking his medication regularly, and states that his condition has fully improved and he has finally been able to get back to doing the things he loves.

CBC with differential	Count	Reference
WBC	6.4 × 103/uL	4–10.5
RBC	5.12 × 106/uL	4.5–5.9
HGB	15.4 g/dL	13.5–17.5
HCT	46%	41%–53%
MCV	90 fL	80–100
MCH	30 pg	27–33
MCHC	33.5 g/dL	32–36
RDW	12.8%	11.5–14.5
Platelets	265 × 103/uL	150–400
Neutrophils	58%	40%–75%
Lymphocytes	30%	20%–45%
Monocytes	8%	2%–10%
Eosinophils	3%	1%–6%
Basophils	1%	0%–2%
BMP		
Sodium	139 mEq/L	135–145
Potassium	4.2 mEq/L	3.5–5.5
Chloride	103 mEq/L	98–107
Bicarbonate	25 mEq/L	22–29
BUN	14 mg/dL	7–20
Creatinine	0.96 mg/dL	0.7–1.3
Glucose	94 mg/dL	70–100
Calcium	9.4 mg/dL	8.5–10.5

CBC with differential	Count	Reference
TSH/Free T4		
TSH	1.8 uIU/mL	0.4–4.0
Free T4	1.2 ng/dL	0.8–1.8
AchR antibodies		
AchR-Binding Ab	12.4 nmol/L (strongly positive)	<0.5 nmol/L
AchR-Blocking Ab	42% inhibition (positive)	<15%
AchR-Modulating Ab	78% loss of receptors (positive)	<20%

Chapter 29

Cardiovascular System: Case 4

Onset	Dizziness was first noticed in her high school junior year approximately 2 weeks after undergoing an exploratory surgery for endometriosis in November 2020. Symptoms are experienced systemically, affecting the entire body.
Location	
Duration	Episodes typically last 5 minutes up to 2 hours.
Characteristics	Episodes of tachycardia with rapid, forceful palpitations. She often felt like her heart is "coming out of her chest" and beyond her control. These episodes are accompanied by shortness of breath after intense physical exertion. She also experienced severe dizziness, beginning with a spinning sensation, progressing to visual disturbances described as "seeing stars" and frequently culminating in syncope. Associated symptoms include nausea, generalized muscle weakness (most prominent in the lower extremities), and profound fatigue, often requiring extended sleep for recovery.
Alleviating/aggravating factors	Alleviating: Light exercise, stress reduction, and elevating her legs to improve cerebral blood flow. Aggravating: Heat exposure is the most severe trigger, Stress
Timing	
Severity	8/10 (varies between 6 and 10)

The patient is 21-year-old White female. Symptom severity and duration vary with activity and stress levels.

On physically demanding or stressful days, symptoms are prolonged and more intense. Conversely, on calm, low-stress days, she may experience only mild symptoms or remain asymptomatic.

Diagnostic Tests:

Electrocardiogram (ECG)

Cardiac monitoring (continuous for 2 months with vital checks)

Magnetic resonance imaging (MRI)

Electroencephalogram (EEG)

Orthostatic testing: The patient was evaluated in supine, seated, and standing positions to monitor changes in HR and BP for concerning trends

Tilt Table Test

Differential Diagnosis:

Orthostatic hypotension

Adrenal insufficiency

Chronic fatigue syndrome

Cardiac arrhythmias

Postural orthostatic tachycardia syndrome (POTS)

Treatment:

Medications:

- Effective: Propranolol, Vitassium C (iron + vitamin C), and salt tablets
- Ineffective: Metoprolol (discontinued due to excessive hypotension)
- Dietary recommendations: Increased sodium intake
- Lifestyle modifications: Incorporation of regular exercise

Chapter 30

Circulatory System: Case 3

Onset	The patient was taken to emergency room by her family after a fall.
Location	
Duration	More than 24 hours.
Characteristics	The patient was weak with irregular heart rhythms prior to the last visit for over 24 hours. Her legs had purpura/bruising. The patient also experienced an eye infection and an ear infection, which required antibiotics.
Alleviating/aggravating factors	NA.
Timing	NA.
Severity	Severe.

An 86-year-old female patient had a mild medical history including COPD and atrial fibrillation. Since 2022, the patient had COPD/emphysema but was controlled.

The patient experienced a fall in early June 2025. Following the fall, she was taken to the emergency room by her family. This initial incident triggered a cascade of subsequent health complications. The patient experienced signs of food poisoning, which led her to no food intake for almost 7 days while taking little fluids. The patient experienced three hospital stays in a month. She had pain in different locations during these three visits. The first visit was the result of a fainting spell brought on by anemia, and she was admitted to Advent Health in Eustis, Florida. For the second visit, the patient had anemia with a failing liver function and atrial fibrillation. The third visit was to Birmingham, Alabama resulting from atrial fibrillation with rapid ventricular responses (RVRs).

In late June 2025, doctors felt she had a gastrointestinal bleed and ceased use of aspirin and blood thinners. In early July 2025, deep vein thrombosis was found in several places in her lower legs. The patient had liver cirrhosis with long standing hypertension and atrial fibrillation. She had macrocytic anemia. Other conditions included macular degeneration, diverticulosis, mild cognitive impairment (the Saint Louis University Mental Status score: 21).

Social history: She was an accountant working at a doctor's office for about 20 years. She retired about 20 years ago and has participated in multiple social clubs and church activities. The patient quit smoking more than 10 years ago. She would consume 4-oz Coca-Cola about four to five times weekly. No illicit or recreational drug use.

Family history: The patient's mother had hypertension and died at in her 60s

Physical Examination:

Purpura/bruising with edema were seen in her legs.

CT scans, ultrasound, and multiple blood tests

Hemoglobin levels (normal range: 12–16):

- 11.7 (12/24/2024)
- 9.7 (4/22/2025)
- 8.1 (6/11/2025)
- 7.3 (6/25/2025)
- 8.6 (7/6/2025)
- 10.8 (9/7/2025)

Name	Value	Previous	Units	Reference range	Flag
WBC	5.98	6.36	10^3/uL	4.1–10.9	Normal
RBC	2.18		10^6/uL	4.2–6.3	Low
HGB	7.6	8.5	g/dL	12–18	Low
HCT	23.7	26.1	%	37–51	Low
MCV	108.7		fL	80–97	High
MCH	34.9		pg	26–32	High
MCHC	32.1		g/dL	31–36	Normal
Platelets	139	133	10^3/uL	140–440	Low
Neutrophils %	31		%	37–92	Low
Lymphocytes %	43.8		%	10–58.5	Normal
Monocytes %	20.4		%	5.5–11.7	High
Eosinophils %	0.2		%	0–2	Normal
Basophils %	1.3		%	0–1.2	Slightly high
Neutrophils #	1.85	2.13	10^3/uL		
Lymphocytes #	2.62		10^3/uL	2–7.8	Low
Monocytes #	1.22		10^3/uL	0.3–0.8	Normal
Eosinophils #	0.01		10^3/uL	0.9–2.9	Low
Basophils #	0.08		10^3/uL	0–0.1	Normal
Gran #	0.2		%	0.00	Normal
RDW-SD	53.8		fL	35.1–43.9	High
RDW (Ratio)	13.4		%	11.5–14.5	Normal

Name	Value	Previous	Units	Reference range	Flag
MPV	11.2		fL	0–49.9	Normal

October 2025:
- Blood pressure: 151/72 mm Hg; heart rate: 86/min; O_2 saturation: 97%; temperature: 98.3; HGB: 8.5

November 2025:
- Checked for viral hepatitis and myelodysplasia
- Bone marrow biopsy

December 2025:
- Myelodysplastic syndrome was diagnosed with bone marrow biopsy

Treatment:

Surgery: Due to numerous clots in legs, an inferior Vana Cava (IVC) filter was put on 7/9/2025.

Medications:
- Metoprolol: 25 mg/once daily
- Losartan: 50 mg/once daily
- Furosemide: 20 mg/once daily
- Pantoprazole: 40 mg/once daily
- Melatonin: 5 mg/once daily
- Lactulose: 10 g/mL once daily
- Senna: 8.6 mg as needed

Diet recommendation(s):
- Heart-healthy diet: High fiber, rich protein, low fat, and low cholesterol

The patient attended inpatient rehabilitation and continued with physical therapy for almost 5 weeks, following which she improved her leg conditions and anemia along with a better diet. Since participating in physical therapy, the patient walks approximately 0.1–0.5 miles daily.

Chapter 31

Circulatory System: Case 4

Onset	Epistaxis and anemia are chronic.
Location	Nose, skin, lungs, and gastrointestinal tract.
Duration	Starting at age 7.
Characteristics	Epistaxis episodes occur without significant discomfort. Anemia leads to fatigue and dyspnea with vigorous activities.
Alleviating/aggravating factors	Afrin is used for intense epistaxis; dry air, high humidity, excitement, and physical contact to the nose are risk factors for epistaxis.
Timing	Sleeping and morning (showers) for epistaxis.
Severity	6 on a scale of 1–10.

The patient is a 49-year-old White female. She quit smoking more than 10 years ago. The patient had pulmonary arteriovenous malformations (AVMs), which are responsible for shortness of breath and double vision. If untreated, these can increase the risk of stroke due to abnormal shunting of blood.

Physical Examination:

Telangiectasias are visible on the ears, tongue, and skin; AVMs were present within nasal passages.

Diagnostic Tests:

CBC, iron studies, and a hereditary hemorrhagic telangiectasia (HHT) panel for genetics
Ultrasound (liver), MRI (brain), bubble echocardiogram (for shunting), CT (lungs, liver, and GI tract)

Treatment:

Medications:

Vitron C: 65 mg twice a day
Rose geranium oil: two sprays each nostril twice a day
Warfarin: 10 mg during treatment of pulmonary AVMs.

Surgical/procedural:
Embolization of pulmonary AVMs

Lifestyle/diet recommendations:
Iron-rich foods, avoids NSAIDs

HHT, also known as Osler-Weber-Rendu disease, is a rare genetic condition affecting blood vessel formation throughout the body. Due to gene mutations, patients develop abnormal dilations and tangles between veins and arteries called telangiectasias or AVMs. It is inherited in a dominant pattern. These malformations can occur anywhere in the body and lead to recurrent bleeding, anemia, and organ complications. Although HHT is a chronic condition, it is manageable with proper monitoring and treatment. Patient education is essential for teaching individuals to recognize early symptoms and enables necessary intervention to reduce long-term risks.

Chapter 32

Infectious Disease: Case 2

Onset	A rash started in 2015.
Location	The rash appeared on the left mid-back extending toward the left side of the chest.
Duration	Symptoms got worse over 1 week.
Characteristics	A red, patchy rash appeared first, then developed into clustered fluid-filled vesicles. The associated pain is sharp and burning. The rash is itchy. The most intense pain was reported in the back, with the front being less severe.
Alleviating/aggravating factors	The pain is worsened by wearing a bra or tight clothing, physical pressure, or contact movement. The pain is alleviated by antiviral medication and minimizing contact, loose clothing, or good rest.
Radiation/related symptoms	None.
Timing	Constant pain became especially severe before treatment and slowly subsided after the treatment was initiated.
Severity	Pain rated as 10/10.

For the first several days, mild irritation (itchy, red rash) began and was thought by the patient to be caused by wearing a bra. One week later, the symptoms got worse. The patient was not be able to sleep or wear normal clothing, which prompted a clinical visit. The associated pain was rated 10/10 at its peak and was described as unbearable burning and stabbing.

Physical Exam:

A unilateral vesicular rash was noted extending from left mid-back to left front chest. Clustered vesicles were fluid-filled and surrounded by inflamed red skin. Gentle palpation revealed high sensitivity in the back region. The rash was seen on one side of the body and followed a clear dermatomal distribution. The pain is sharp and burning. No sensory loss or motor weakness was seen in the same area. No systemic symptoms such as fever, fatigue, or malaise were reported.

A clinical diagnosis was made based solely on the physical exam and history of clinical symptoms. No lab tests or cultures were performed.

Past medical history:

Varicella infection (chickenpox) as a child. Does not have a history of immunosuppression or chronic illnesses.

Treatment:

Oral antiviral medication: Valacyclovir initiated promptly after the diagnosis of shingles was made. No topical creams or pain medications were prescribed.

Rash and symptoms improved gradually. A complete healing occurred over several months and no residual scaring left.

Lifestyle changes: Wore loose clothing and avoided physical contact with rash. Advised to monitor for worsening pain or new symptoms. The patient was in her early 30s, which is atypical for shingles, making the case a rare presentation in an otherwise healthy adult. The patient probably developed shingles due to stress, overwork, and an unhealthy lifestyle. Besides maintaining a work/life balance, the patient was also advised to have a healthy diet.

Prevention:

Shingrix vaccine is a preventive option for older adults. However, it is not for this patient for her young age (below 50).

Chapter 33

Nervous System: Case 4

Onset	Excessive daytime sleepiness (EDS) and sleep attacks began around age 11, with cataplexy and hallucinations starting around age 14. Autonomic behavior began around age 15. The patient is currently 22 years old.
Location	Many symptoms are either mental or systemic. For cataplexy, knees and arms were commonly affected, though full-body collapses were seen during stress or exertion.
Duration	Narcolepsy is chronic with symptoms fluctuating with severity but is not fully resolved. Sleep attacks and cataplexy can be brief or extended with re-triggers (recurrence).
Characteristics	Symptoms include overwhelming fatigue, sudden sleep attacks, vivid hallucinations, cataplexy, and autonomic behaviors.
Alleviating factors	Rest, strict sleep schedule, scheduled naps, medication.
Aggravating factors	Stress, insufficient sleep, dietary changes, physical exertion, caffeine, hormonal shifts, vaccines, sudden emotional shifts, medication adjustments, daylight saving time change, prolonged inactivity, laughter (specifically triggers cataplexy), and emotional instability.
Timing	Sleep attacks are most severe at 8–10 a.m.; 2–4 p.m. Symptoms of EDS and fatigue worsen from waking to the next sleep period. Disturbed sleep occurs at night. Most symptoms occur around the time to sleep.
Severity	The patient scores 13/24 on the Epworth Sleepiness Scale with medication, and 18 without. Cataplexy varies from monthly to daily. Hallucinations occur at least twice weekly. Sleep attacks happen from daily to monthly depending on external factors.

Cataplexy is a symptom of narcolepsy type I and can be defined as a sudden and uncontrollable, brief loss of muscle tone. In patients with narcolepsy, this is often caused by experiencing strong or intense emotions. It can range from partial cataplexy to full cataplexy, which is different in everyone. Examples include slurred speech, weakness of the face, limbs, and trunk, resulting in slumping to ground and unable to move or talk.

Cataplexy occurs several times a month when medicated or several times a day unmedicated. Hallucinations occur at minimum twice a week to a degree where the patient is so disoriented that reality does not align with the hallucination upon waking. Disrupted sleep is rare when medicated but consistently unmedicated. Sleep attacks range from every day to a few times a month depending on external factors even when medicated, though mostly occurring after 6 p.m. when medicated.

Cataplectic attacks are generally short-lived (a few seconds to 10 minutes). However, for re-triggering episodes, the loss of function can last over an hour in severe cases (a highly atypical presentation). Sleep attacks typically last between 10 and 30 minutes, unless the patient is stressed or overexerted, in which case the sleep attack may either (1) last several hours; or (2) retrigger (the patient has recurrent attacks every hour or two). This is typically a stress response and lasts 1 to 4 days.

Excessive daytime sleepiness (EDS) is an overwhelming urge to sleep/inability to stay awake, frequently accompanied by brain fog symptoms, lack of energy, and extreme fatigue.

Sleep attacks are when the body "shuts down" and the patient is physically incapable of not falling asleep, typically with a rapid onset, though fighting can prolong symptoms before sleep sets in.

Disrupted sleep is when the patient has difficulty staying asleep for prolonged periods of time, typically a few hours.

Cataplexy is a loss of muscle tone, typically in response to strong emotions.

Hypnagogic hallucinations are vivid dream-like experiences as someone is falling asleep or waking up. The hallucinations can involve all senses, though visual, auditory, and tactile are most common. The patient has all three main types of hallucinations, but she also experiences smell and pain in some cases.

Autonomic behavior is when a person does things without full awareness or conscious control, frequently when fighting sleepiness, falling asleep, or while asleep, without a memory of these actions. The patient experiences all three to varying degrees with fighting sleepiness having the most notable severity as the patient is the most "conscious" at that stage and is unaware that she is past the point of normal cognitive functioning.

Family history: Positive

Social history: The patient is homeschooled.

Physical Examination:

The patient was diagnosed using overnight sleep study and a Multiple Sleep Latency Test (MSLT). She was found falling asleep four of the five times and the missed nap was due to an auditory hypnagogic hallucination causing an anxiety spike that prevented sleep in the allotted 15 minutes. While entrances into Rapid Eye Movement (REM) sleep were not consistent with diagnostic criteria, the patient presented with cataplexy and admitted to accidentally taking her extended-release attention-deficit/hyperactivity disorder (ADHD) stimulant medication in the morning of the test which is known to be able to hinder sleep and entering REM.

Narcolepsy was diagnosed using: (1) Overnight sleep study and a MSLT; (2) How often REM sleep is entered and how quickly it is entered; (3) Presence of cataplexy; (4) Epworth Sleepiness Scale

Treatment:

Medication: The patient trialed multiple stimulant medications but reacted poorly to them. Xywave and Xyrem reduced symptoms but caused severe nausea and rapid weight loss (50 lbs in 3 months, including 11 lbs in 5 days). A daytime dose of Wakix (a histamine inducer) was used to keep her awake and a nightly tablet of muscle relaxer Baclofen helps her sleep through the night.

Lifestyle changes: Sticking to a set sleep schedule is also part of the plan, even though school demands make it hard. Because narcolepsy can slow down metabolism and raise the risk of developing diabetes, she has been recommended to be careful of her sugar intake. Together, all these control her daytime drowsiness while helping her long-term overall health.

The Epworth sleepiness scale is a tool used to examine the degree of a person's daytime sleepiness.

The results of the scale range from 0 to 24. Results that fall between 0 and 10 show average (normal) daytime sleepiness. A score under 10 is not necessarily a cause for concern, but it could indicate. A score between 11 and 24 tends to indicate excessive (abnormal) daytime sleepiness.

- 0 to 5: Low daytime sleepiness (normal).
- 6 to 10: High daytime sleepiness (normal).
- 11 to 12: Mild excessive daytime sleepiness.
- 13 to 15: Moderate excessive daytime sleepiness.
- 16 to 24: Severe excessive daytime sleepiness.

Epworth Sleepiness Scale

How likely are you to doze off or fall asleep in the following situations?

Use the following scale to choose the most appropriate number:

0 **No chance**	**1** **Slight chance**	**2** **Moderate chance**	**3** **High chance**	
Sitting and reading	0	1	2	3
Watching television	0	1	2	3
Sitting inactive, in a public space	0	1	2	3
Lying down to rest in the afternoon when circumstances permit	0	1	2	3
Sitting and talking to someone	0	1	2	3
Sitting quietly after lunch without alcohol	0	1	2	3
As a passenger in car for an hour without a break	0	1	2	3
In a car, while stopped for a few minutes in traffic	0	1	2	3
	Total score:			

Chapter 34

Nervous System: Case 5

Onset	Sudden, severe left-sided posterior occipital pain on October 17, 2010.
Location	Left posterior occipital region.
Duration	Initial episode lasted for about 45 minutes; persistent and recurrent thereafter.
Characteristics	Sharp.
Alleviating factors	Acupuncture.
Aggravating factors	None.
Timing	Sudden onset while preparing breakfast; ongoing afterward.
Severity	Severe (10/10).

The patient is a 45-year-old female, who served in the United States Air Force (U.S.A.F). The patient had a history of migraines due to viral meningitis in 2009. On October 17, 2010, the patient had a sudden episode of severe, sharp left-sided posterior occipital pain. She was in the kitchen preparing breakfast for her two children when the pain began. She dropped to her knees with the pain being 10/10. The pain dulled after 45 minutes. On October 18, 2010, she received acupuncture and intramuscular Toradol, which were ineffective. On October 19, 2010, she received a head CT that showed a possible subdural hematoma and was then transferred to the hospital. Besides severe occipital headaches, the patient had left thumb numbness/weakness, nausea, decreased appetite, and constipation. The patients also lost 27 pounds of body weight. She was unable to work sometimes.

Possible diagnoses:

- Subdural hematoma
- Subarachnoid hemorrhage

- Cervical artery dissection
- Occipital neuralgia
- Tension headache or migraine

Physical Examination:

Initial head CT (November 2010): Possible subdural hematoma

Repeat CT (January 2011): C2–C3 degenerative disc osteophyte complex; C4–C5 degenerative disc osteophyte complex; C5–C6 disc herniation; C6–C7 small central broad-based disc protrusion

Treatment:

The patient underwent a C5–C6 anterior cervical discectomy with fusion. The pain did not resolve, and other symptoms still existed. First surgery was performed in April 2011; medications were initiated in May 2011; a spinal cord stimulator was placed posteriorly and ran down the spine for the charger port on the left posterior hip in September 2011.

Persistence of chronic neuropathic pain despite anterior cervical discectomy and fusion (ACDF) surgery and multimodal pain management; daily function and quality of life were impacted; once spinal cord surgery was complete, the medication oxycodone and fentanyl subsided due to therapy and pain patches. She went to physical therapy and pain clinic on a consistent basis, and the following medications were given:

Lyrica 75 mg po QHS
IV IR (quick release oxycontin)
Fentanyl patch 25 mcg change q 72 hours
Sennekot QHS
Colace 100 mg po BID
Effexor 37.5 mg po BID
Vitamin B-12 injections q week then q month

Chapter 35

Inflammation: Case 2

Onset	Symptoms began at age 19, approximately 3 months following a COVID-19 infection.
Location	Lower back; sacroiliac joint.
Duration	Ongoing for 3 years.
Characteristics	Persistent chronic back pain; sacroiliac joint tenderness and reduced spinal mobility; fatigue.
Alleviating factors	Physical activity.
Aggravating factors	Prolonged rest or inactivity, overexertion, stress, and fatigue
Timing	Nocturnal pain, particularly in the second half of the night; Morning stiffness, lasting longer than 30 minutes
Severity	

Non-radiographic axial spondyloarthritis is a form of chronic inflammatory arthritis that primarily affects the spine and sacroiliac joints. It falls under the broad category of axial spondyloarthritis, which includes both non-radiographic axial spondyloarthritis and ankylosing spondylitis.

Unlike ankylosing spondylitis, non-radiographic axial spondyloarthritis does not present visible structural damage on standard X-rays. However, it can still cause significant inflammation detectable by MRI. Both conditions share common features including chronic back pain, morning stiffness, fatigue, and reduced spinal mobility.

Non-radiographic axial spondyloarthritis typically begins in early adulthood, most often between late teens and early 30s although it can start later in life. Most commonly, symptoms first appear in the lower back or sacroiliac joints. Symptoms usually develop gradually, starting with intermittent lower back pain and stiffness—particularly in the sacroiliac joints, that may worsen over time.

For mild to moderate cases, patients experience manageable levels of pain and stiffness, particularly in the lower back and sacroiliac joints. Symptoms may fluctuate and often improve with physical activity or treatment, allowing individuals to manage the condition well with lifestyle changes and non-steroidal anti-inflammatory drugs (NSAIDs). For severe cases, there is increased pain, stiffness, and fatigue. Functional impairment may occur, with reduced range of motion in the spine and joints, which can affect mobility. Inflammatory flare-ups can result in painful swelling in areas like the knees, hips, or shoulders, further limiting function.

Early diagnosis and appropriate treatment are essential to prevent disease progression and preserve quality of life. If untreated or inadequately managed, the non-radiographic axial spondyloarthritis can progress to radiographic axial spondyloarthritis, resulting in structural joint damage and, in severe cases, ankylosis (spinal fusion), leading to significant loss of mobility.

Aggravating factors:

- Rest or inactivity: Symptoms often worsen with prolonged inactivity, such as sleeping or sitting for long periods (this is called *inflammatory back pain*).
- Early morning hours: Pain and stiffness are typically worse in the morning upon waking.
- Cold or damp weather: Some patients report worsening symptoms in cold, wet environments.
- Stress or fatigue: Emotional or physical stress and poor sleep may aggravate symptoms.
- Physical overexertion: Although moderate activity helps, excessive or improper exercise can worsen pain.

Alleviating factors:

- Physical activity and exercise: Movement often reduces stiffness and pain, especially low-impact activities like walking, swimming, or yoga.
- Warmth or heat therapy: Warm showers, baths, or heating pads can help relieve stiffness and discomfort.
- Anti-inflammatory medications (NSAIDs): These are often effective in reducing inflammation and pain.
- Stretching and physical therapy: Targeted exercises can improve flexibility and spinal mobility.
- Good sleep posture and ergonomic support: Supportive mattresses or chairs can help reduce strain on the back and joints.

Physical Examination:

Reduced spinal mobility, particularly in the lumbar region; positive response to NSAIDs, consistent with inflammatory etiology; bilateral sacroiliac joint tenderness, with a positive FABER test on the left; widespread joint tenderness, including multiple metacarpophalangeal (MCP) joints, metatarsophalangeal (MTP) joints, and bilateral ankle/Achilles regions; associated symptoms include brittle nails, tendonitis, and enthesitis, painful lower back and spinal tenderness on palpation, pain, and stiffness in the hands.

Note: The FABER (Patrick's) test, stands for: Flexion, Abduction and External Rotation, is a clinical pain provocation test designed to assist in diagnosis of pathologies in the hip, lumbar spine, and sacroiliac.

Laboratory findings:

- HLA-B27: Negative
- Inflammatory markers (ESR, CRP): Within normal range
- Rheumatoid factor: Elevated
- Sarcoiliac joints (X-ray/MRI): Normal
- X-ray of the lumbar and thoracic spine reveals mild scoliosis
- MRI of the lumbar spine shows minor degenerative changes and confirms mild scoliosis
- X-rays of hands and feet show severe joint deterioration, particularly in small joints

Treatment:

The patient initially experienced a marked reduction in stiffness with Celecoxib (Celebrex), indicating a positive response to NSAIDs.

The patient was started on adalimumab (Humira) and reported significant symptom relief following the initial dose. However, subsequent doses (second and third) failed to sustain therapeutic benefit.

Therapy was transitioned to secukinumab (Cosentyx). The patient reported substantial symptom relief during the loading phase (150 mg weekly for 5 weeks) and the first maintenance dose (150 mg/month) and then slowly began feeling more pain towards each maintenance dose (days of pain increasing with each dose). Patient is currently being treated with 300 mg Cosentyx pen (once a month) and Celebrex.

Chapter 36

Endocrine System: Case 4

Onset	Unknown weight gain since May 2022
Location	Thyroid gland
Duration	2 years
Characteristics	Weight gain, increased resting heart rate, enlarged thyroid gland
Alleviating factors	
Aggravating factors	Food with gluten or dairy, intense exercise, lack of sleep, caffeine, stress
Timing	
Severity	

The 20-year-old White female is highly active (DOB: 12/16/2002). She has a history of an elevated body mass index (BMI) but recently lost a significant amount of weight before seeking treatment. While training for a half-marathon, the patient experienced a significant increase in resting heart rate, weight, and fatigue prompting her to seek a medical visit. She has no notable medical history. She has no family history of Hashimoto's disease or hypothyroidism.

BMI: 31.58 (Index)
BP: 126/70 (mm Hg)
HR: 68/min
RR: 16/min
Weight: 184 lbs
Height: 5'4"
ECG: Normal sinus rhythm

August 15, 2023—CBC was ordered with differential and basic metabolic panels. TSH level was elevated.

November 14, 2023—TSH: 7.57 uIU/mL (0.27–4.2); T4: 6.9 ug/dL (4.5–11.7).

November 20, 2023—TSH: 18.5 uIU/mL (0.27–4.2); T4: 6.3 ug/dL (4.5–11.7). Thyroglobulin Ab: 1 IU/mL (< or =1)

BMI: 33.12 (index)
BP: 126/70 mmHg
HR: 72/min
RR: 16/min
Weight: 193 lbs
Height: 5'4"

Other medications:

Taking clindamycin topical: 1%, one app applied two times a day for 30 days
Taking Junel Fe 1/20: 1 mg, one tablet, orally once a day
Taking tretinoin topical: 0.05%, one app applied once a day (at bedtime) for 30 days

February 20, 2024—The patient was taking 25 micrograms of Synthroid daily. TSH: 9.87 uIU/mL (0.27–4.2); T4: 6.9 ug/dL (4.5–11.7). Thyroglobulin Ab: 1 IU/mL (< or = 1); Thyroid Peroxidase Ab: 902 IU/mL (< 9)

BMI: 34.15 (index)
BP: 106/60 mmHg
HR: 88/min
RR: 16/min
Weight: 199 lbs
Height: 5'4"

Other current medications:

Taking clindamycin topical: 1%, one app applied two times a day for 30 days
Taking Junel Fe 1/20: 1 mg, one tablet, orally once a day
Taking tretinoin topical: 0.05% one app applied once a day (at bedtime) for 30 days

March 28, 2024—The patient was taking 50 micrograms of Synthroid daily. T4 and TSH were ordered, which showed lower TSH than the previous visit but still above the normal range. TSH: 9.87 uIU/mL (0.27–4.2); T4: 6.9 ug/dL (4.5–11.7). Thyroglobulin Ab: 1 IU/mL (< or = 1); Thyroid Peroxidase Ab: 902 IU/mL (< 9)

April 2, 2024—T4 and TSH were ordered, which showed lower TSH than the previous visit but still above the normal range. TSH: 8.79 uIU/mL (0.27–4.2); T4: 8.4 ug/dL (4.5–11.7).

BMI: 34.5 (index)
BP: 122/60 mmHg
HR: 88/min
RR: 16/min
Weight: 201 lbs
Height: 5'4"

Start Synthroid: 50 microgram one tablet orally once a day for 30 days; refills: three

Other current medications:

Taking Synthroid: 25 micrograms, one tablet, orally once a day for 30 days; refills: three
Taking clindamycin topical: 1%, one app applied two times a day for 30 days
Taking Junel Fe 1/20: 1 mg, one tablet, orally once a day
Taking tretinoin topical: 0.05%, one app applied once a day (at bedtime) for 30 days

May 14, 2024—The patient was taking 75 micrograms of Synthroid daily. T4 and TSH were ordered, which showed lower TSH than the previous visit but still above the normal range.

BMI: 34.84 (index)
BP: 110/80 mmHg
HR: 64/min

RR: 16/min
Weight: 203 lbs
Height: 5'4"
Start Synthroid: 75 micrograms, one tablet, orally once a day

Other current medications:

Stop Synthroid: 50 micrograms, one tablet, orally once a day
Stop Synthroid: 25 micrograms, one tablet, orally once a day
Taking clindamycin topical: 1%, one app applied two times a day for 30 days
Taking Junel Fe 1/20: 1 mg one tab, orally once a day
Taking tretinoin topical: 0.05%, one app applied once a day (at bedtime) for 30 days

June 21, 2024—T4 and TSH were ordered. TSH: 5.19 uIU/mL (0.27–4.2); T4: 9.5 ug/dL (4.5–11.7). The patient was taking 88 micrograms of Synthroid daily.

June 24, 2024—The patient was taking 88 micrograms of Synthroid daily.
BMI: 34.5 (index)
BP: 118/70 mmHg
HR: 68/min
RR: 16/min
Weight: 201 lbs
Height: 5'4"

Start Synthroid: 88 micrograms, one tablet, orally once a day

Stop Synthroid: 75 micrograms, one tablet, orally once a day

Other medications:

Taking clindamycin topical: 1%, one app applied two times a day for 30 days
Taking Junel Fe 1/20: 1 mg, one tablet, orally once a day
Taking tretinoin topical: 0.05%, one app applied once a day (at bedtime) for 30 days

October 9, 2024—The patient was taking 88 micrograms of Synthroid daily and was stable.
BMI: 33.64 (index)
BP: 118/76 mmHg
HR: 60/min
RR: 16/min
Weight: 196 lbs
Height: 5'4"

Other current medications:

Taking Synthroid: 88 micrograms, one tablet orally once a day for 30 days; refills: five
Taking clindamycin topical: 1%, one app applied two times a day for 30 days
Taking Junel Fe 1/20: 1 mg one tablet, orally once a day
Taking tretinoin topical: 0.05%, one app applied once a day (at bedtime) for 30 days

April 4, 2025—The patient was taking 88 micrograms of Synthroid daily and was asymptomatic.
BMI: 31.07 (index)
BP: 100/70 mmHg
HR: 72/min
RR: 16/min
Weight: 181 lbs
Height: 5'4"

Other current medications:

Taking Synthroid: 88 micrograms, one tablet, orally once a day for 90 days; refills: three
Taking clindamycin topical: 1%, one app applied two times a day for 30 days
Taking Junel Fe 1/20: 1 mg, one tablet, orally once a day

Taking tretinoin topical: 0.05%, one app applied once a day (at bedtime) for 30 days

Over the course of about a year, the dose of Synthroid was adjusted based on the levels of T4 and TSH. The T4 levels fluctuated but never fell out of the normal range. TSH levels were high but decreased along with increased dose of Synthroid. During the course, the patient's body weight fluctuated as well.

While adjusting her medication, she experienced mood swings, disruptions in sleep schedules, and varying energy levels. Her ability to exercise was impacted (for example, fainting with minimal energy exertion). Appetite changed as well. In addition, choosing foods to alleviate symptoms was expensive and time-consuming.

Keep on a dairy-free and gluten free diet, limit caffeine intake, decrease high-intensity exercise, limit stressors, and regulate sleep schedule.

Hashimoto's Thyroiditis

It is also known as chronic lymphocytic thyroiditis or autoimmune thyroiditis, in which the immune system attacks one's own thyroid gland, specifically thyroid peroxidase enzyme (TPO) and thyroglobulin. It is the most common cause of hypothyroidism with inflammation as well as a decreased production of thyroid hormone.

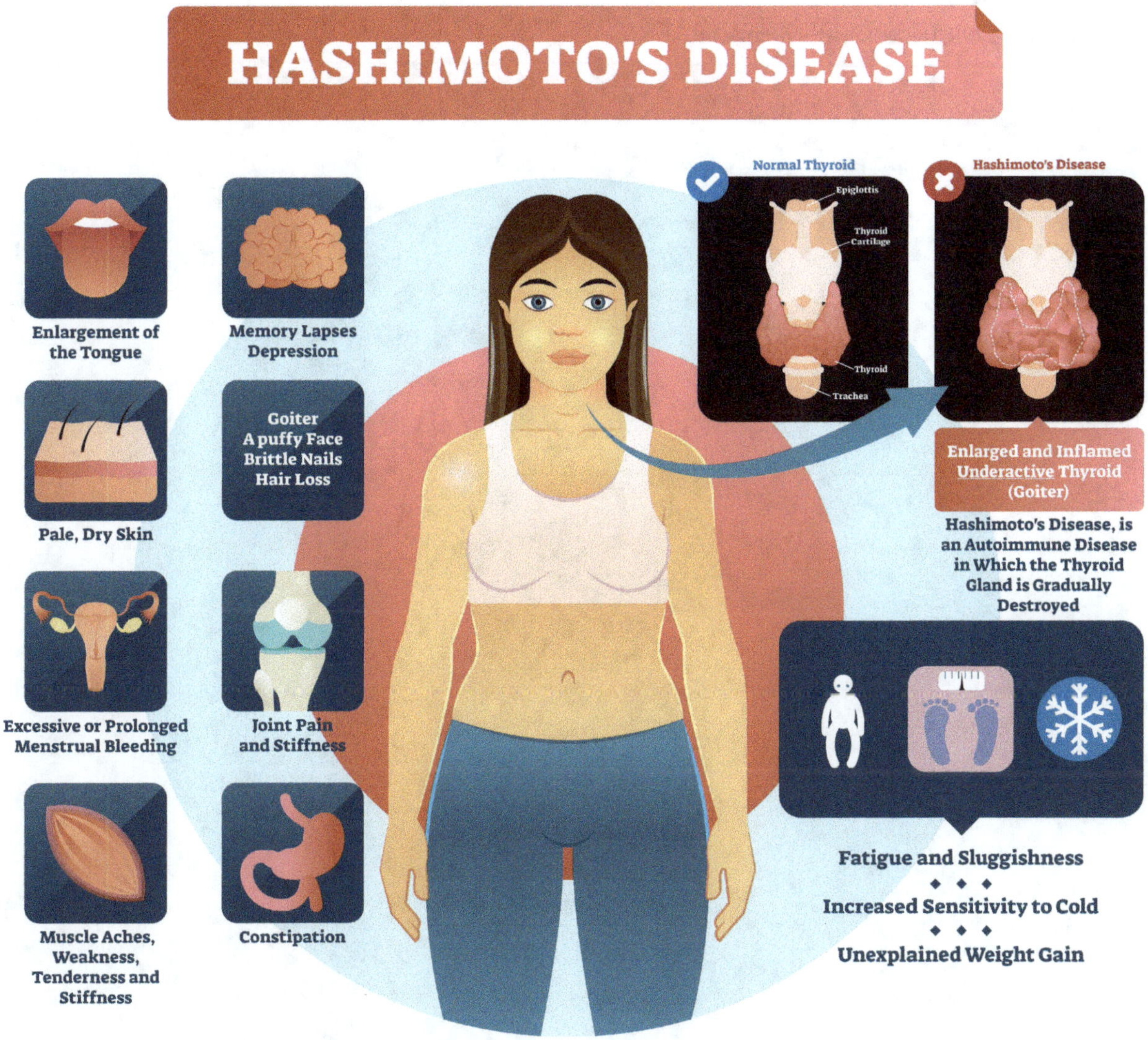

Figure 36.1 Hashimoto's Thyroiditis

Risk factors: Being female, genetics, bacterial infections?

Symptoms: Fatigue, abnormal weight gain, constipation, increased sensitivity to cold, depression, muscle aches, difficulty exercising, irregular or heavy menstrual periods.

General hypothyroidism can be determined by a blood panel showing TSH and T4/T3 levels. It would be indicated by high TSH and low T4/T3 levels. The presence of a goiter often accompanies hypothyroidism due to high TSH levels, which could trigger thyroid growth, producing more surface areas to compensate for low efficiency.

Hashimoto's disease can present all prior evidence, but it is distinguished by positive antibody tests for thyroid peroxidase antibodies and/or thyroglobulin antibodies. An ultrasound can be performed to assess the size of the thyroid and potential scars caused by the autoimmune attacks.

Image Credits

Fig. 36.1: Copyright © 2018 Depositphotos/VectorMine.

Appendix

Common Diagnostic Tests

X-Ray

X-Ray is a form of electromagnetic radiation. X-rays have high energy and can pass through objects in different degrees depending on the composition (density) of the object or different parts of the object including the human body. Medical X-rays are used to generate images of tissues and organs of the body. After X-rays travel through the body part, an X-ray detector picks up the signal and an image will be formed that represents the "shadows" from the part(s) of the body.

One type of X-ray detector is photographic film, but there are many other types of detectors that are used to produce digital images. The X-ray images that result from this process are called radiographs.

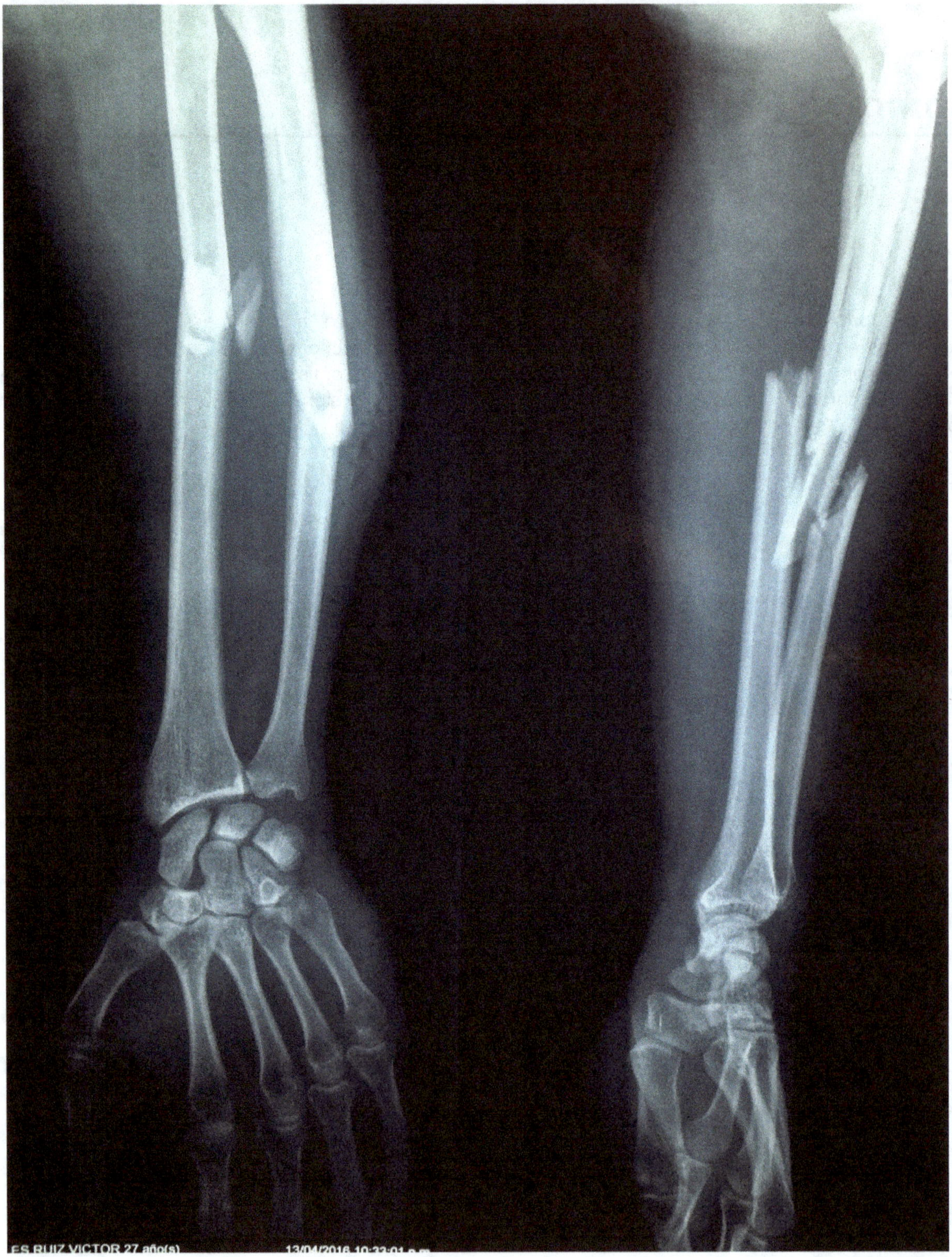

Figure A.1

Mammography

Mammography is radiography used to detect or diagnose breast cancer/tumor. Mammograms can also detect microcalcifications, which show up as bright specks.

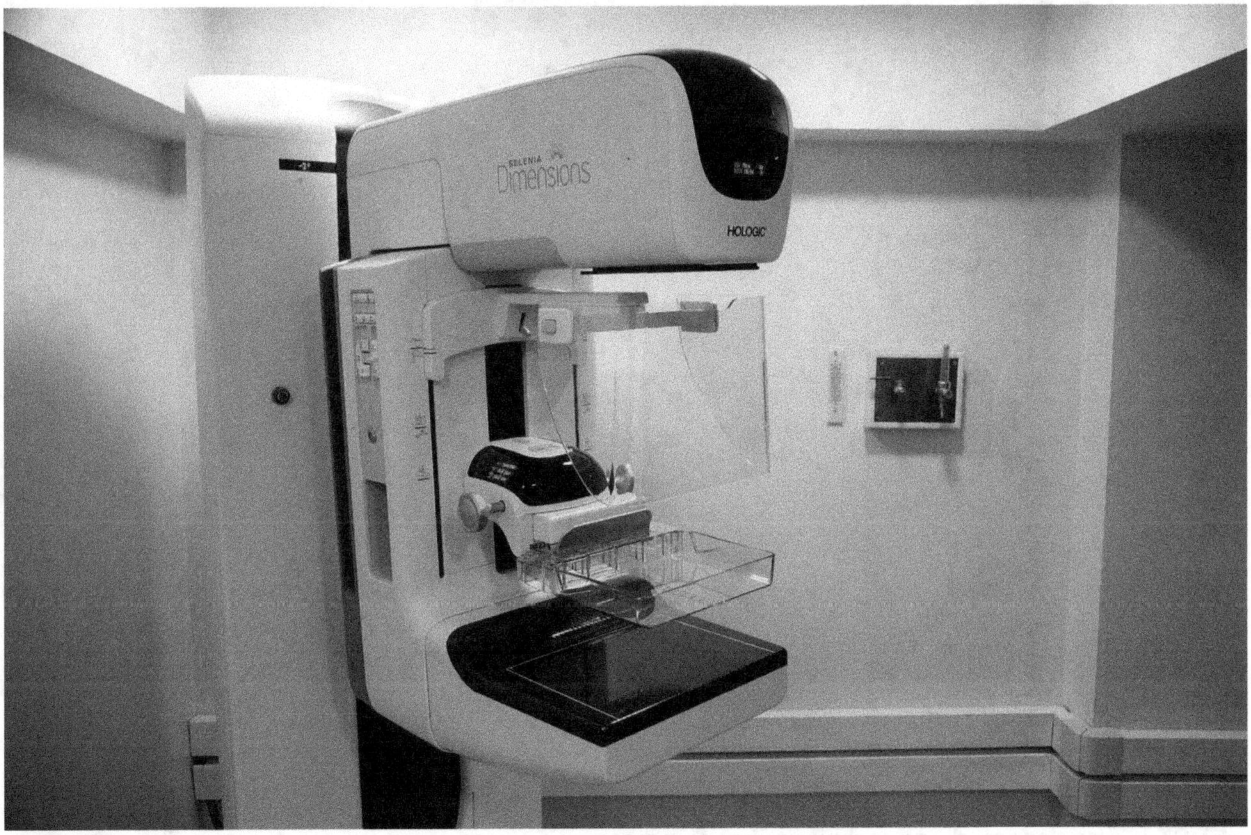

Figure A.2

Computed Tomography (CT)

CT uses a computer to process a series of cross-sectional images of the body. CT images give more details than plain radiographs. Correspondingly, the radiation exposure from CT is more than the plain x-ray.

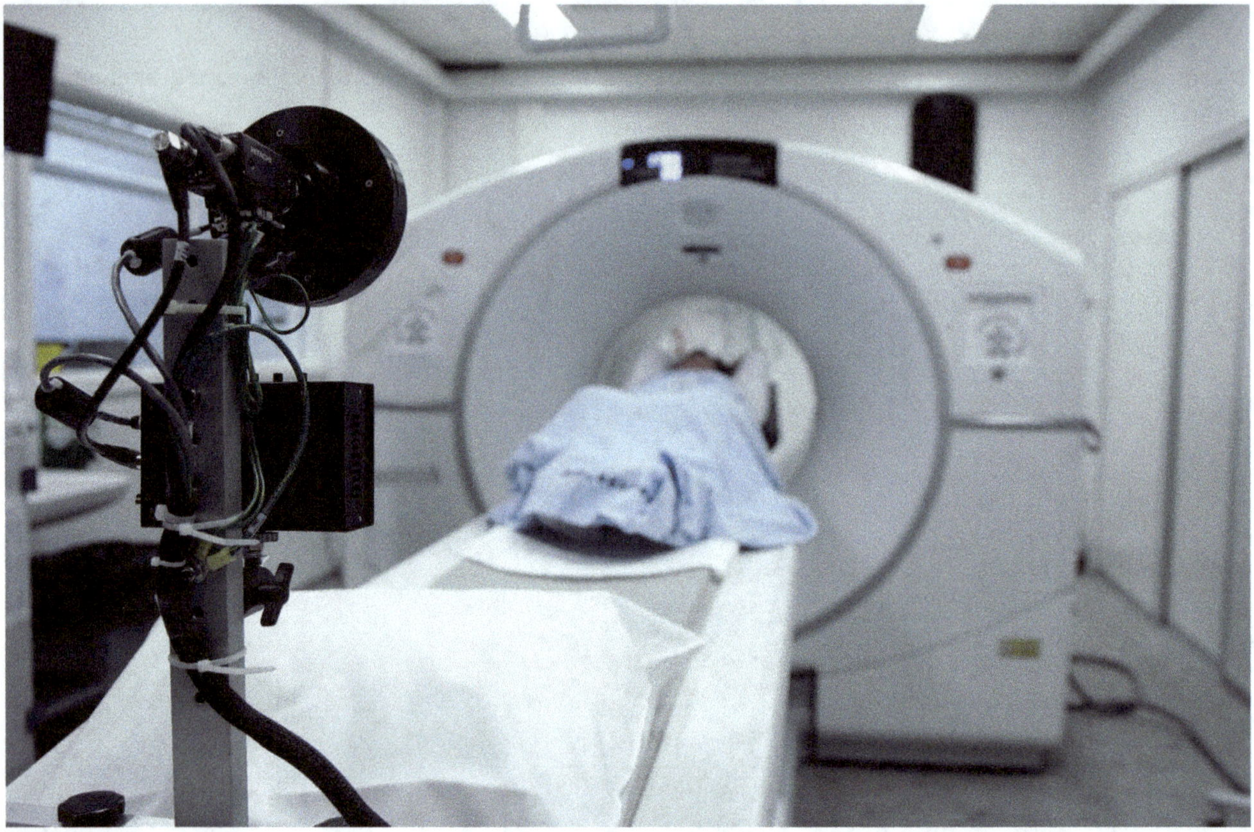

Figure A.3

Positron Emission Tomography (PET)-CT

PET-CT is a nuclear medicine technique that combines a PET scanner and a CT scanner. The image tells the local metabolic activity in a specific body part. It is a commonly used tool to diagnose cancerous formations in the body. Cancer or tumor tissue has higher metabolic activity than normal corresponding tissue.

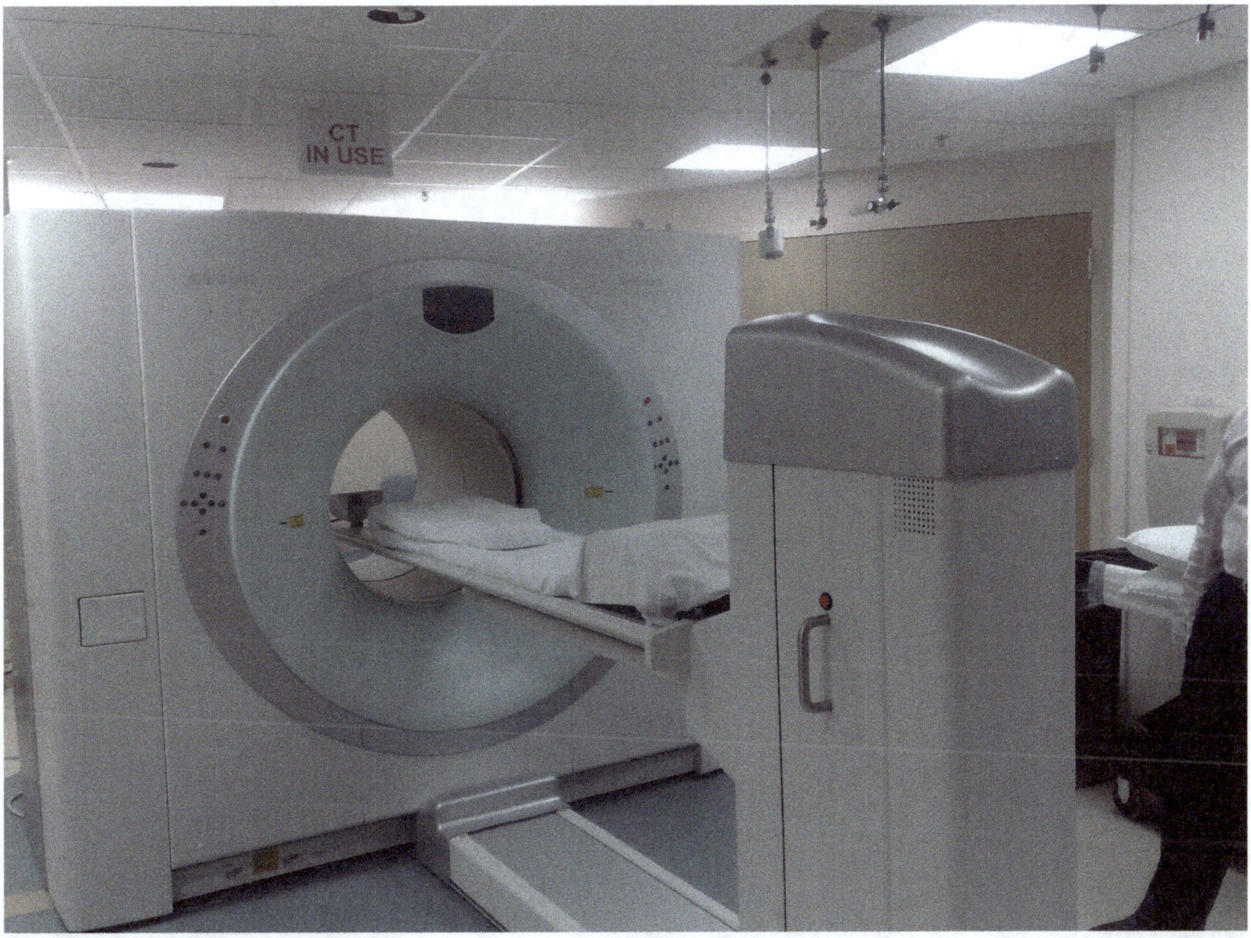

Figure A.4a

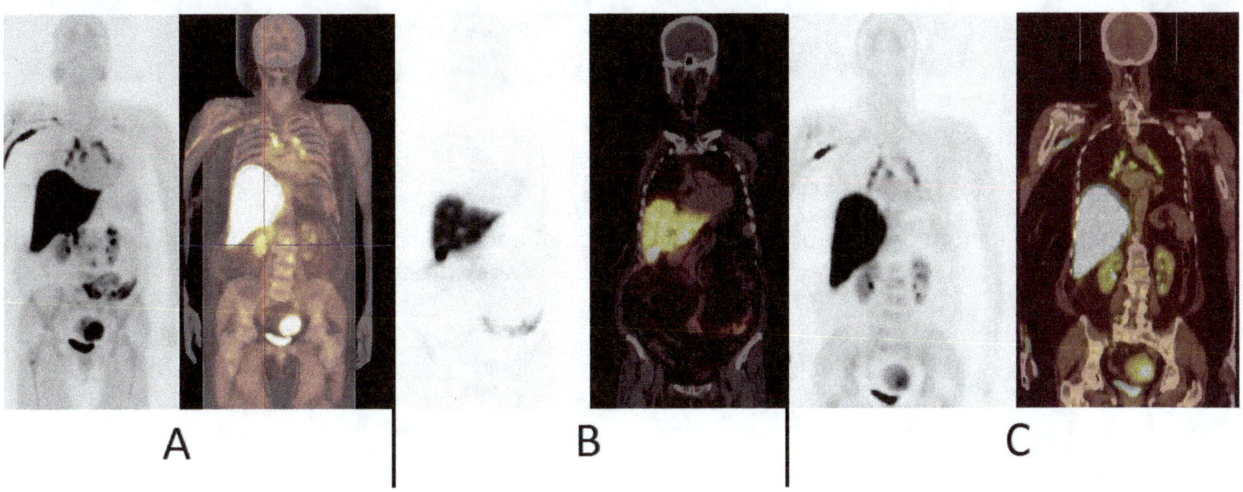

Figure A.4b

Fluoroscopy

Fluoroscopy uses X-ray technology and a fluorescent screen to obtain images of a radiographic contrast agent introduced into the body. For example, fluoroscopy is used to view blood flow to the heart muscle and to see through blood vessels and organs. This technology can also be used to guide an internally threaded catheter during cardiac angioplasty, which is a minimally invasive procedure for opening clogged arteries that supply blood to the heart.

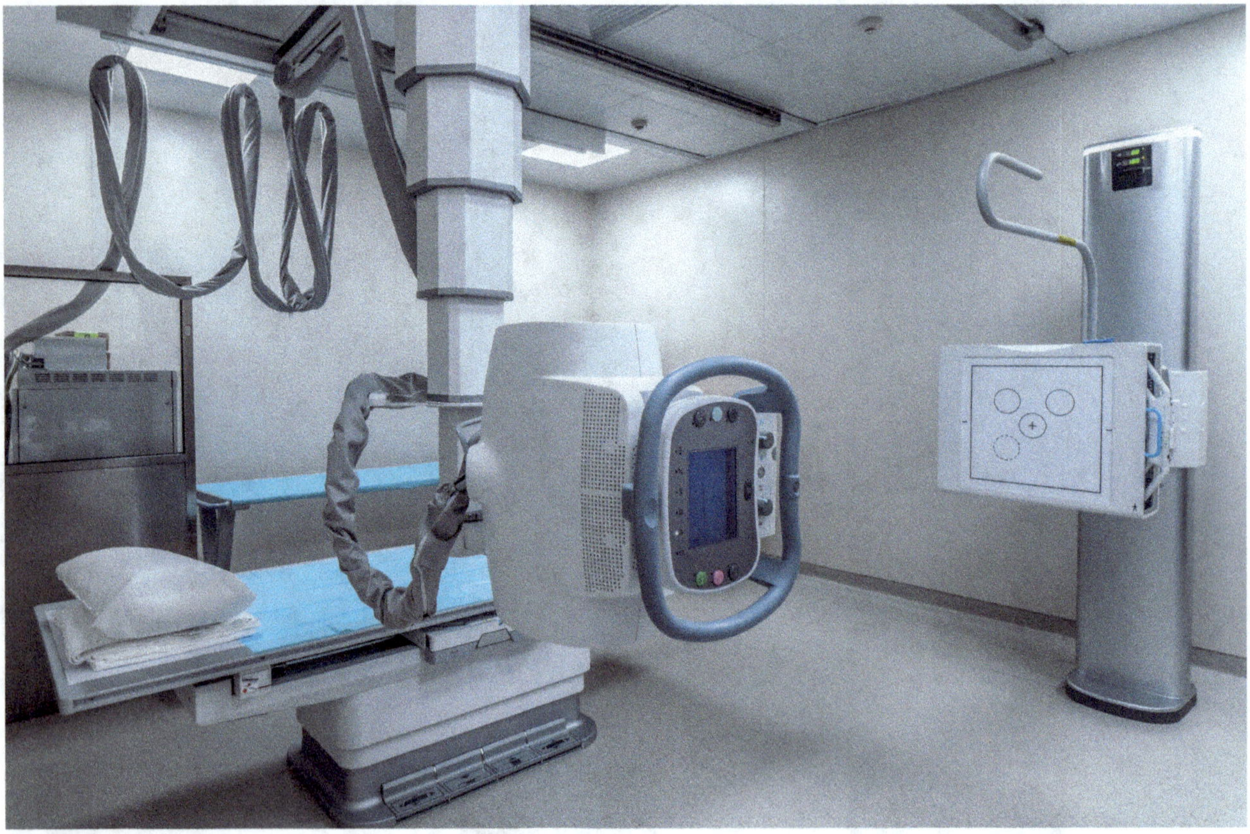

Figure A.5

Magnetic Resonance Imaging (MRI)

MRI is a medical imaging technique used to form pictures of body organs. MRI does not use ionizing radiation; instead, it uses magnets and radio waves to produce images on a computer.

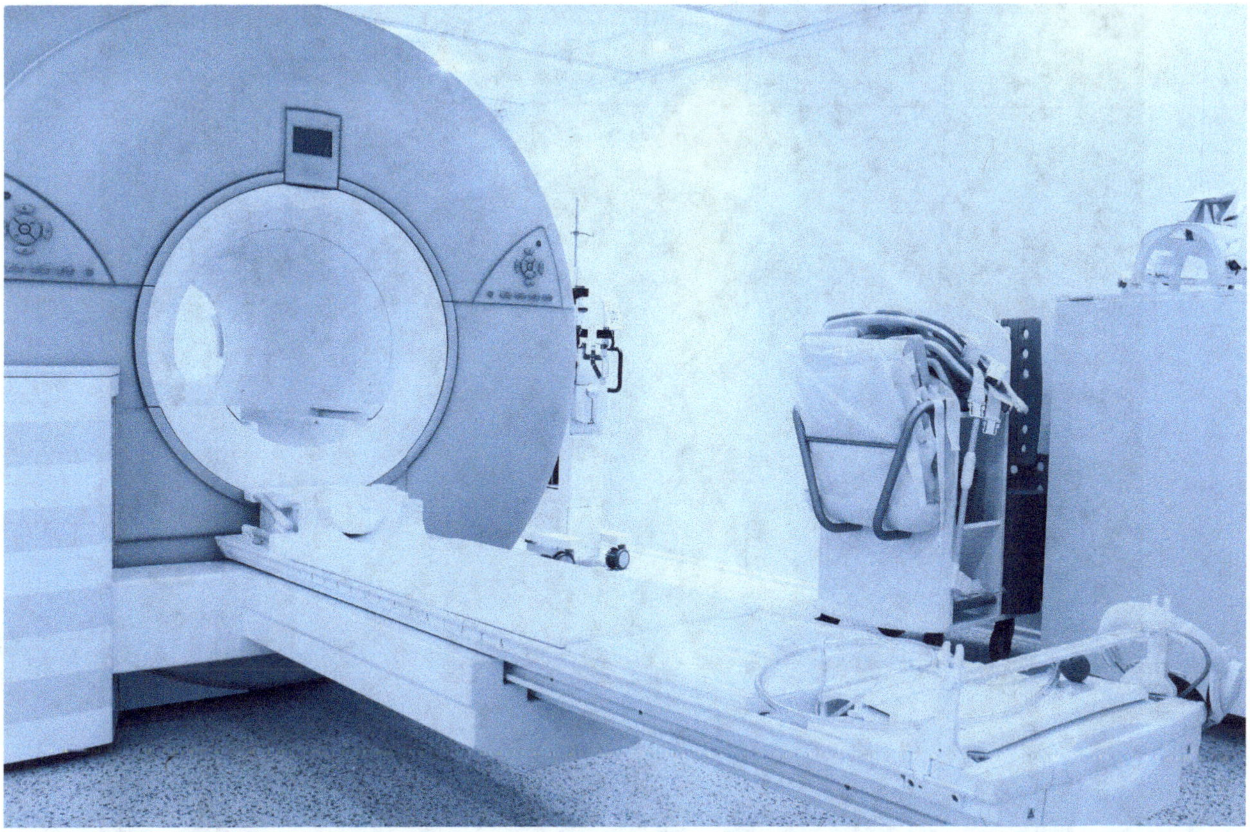

Figure A.6a

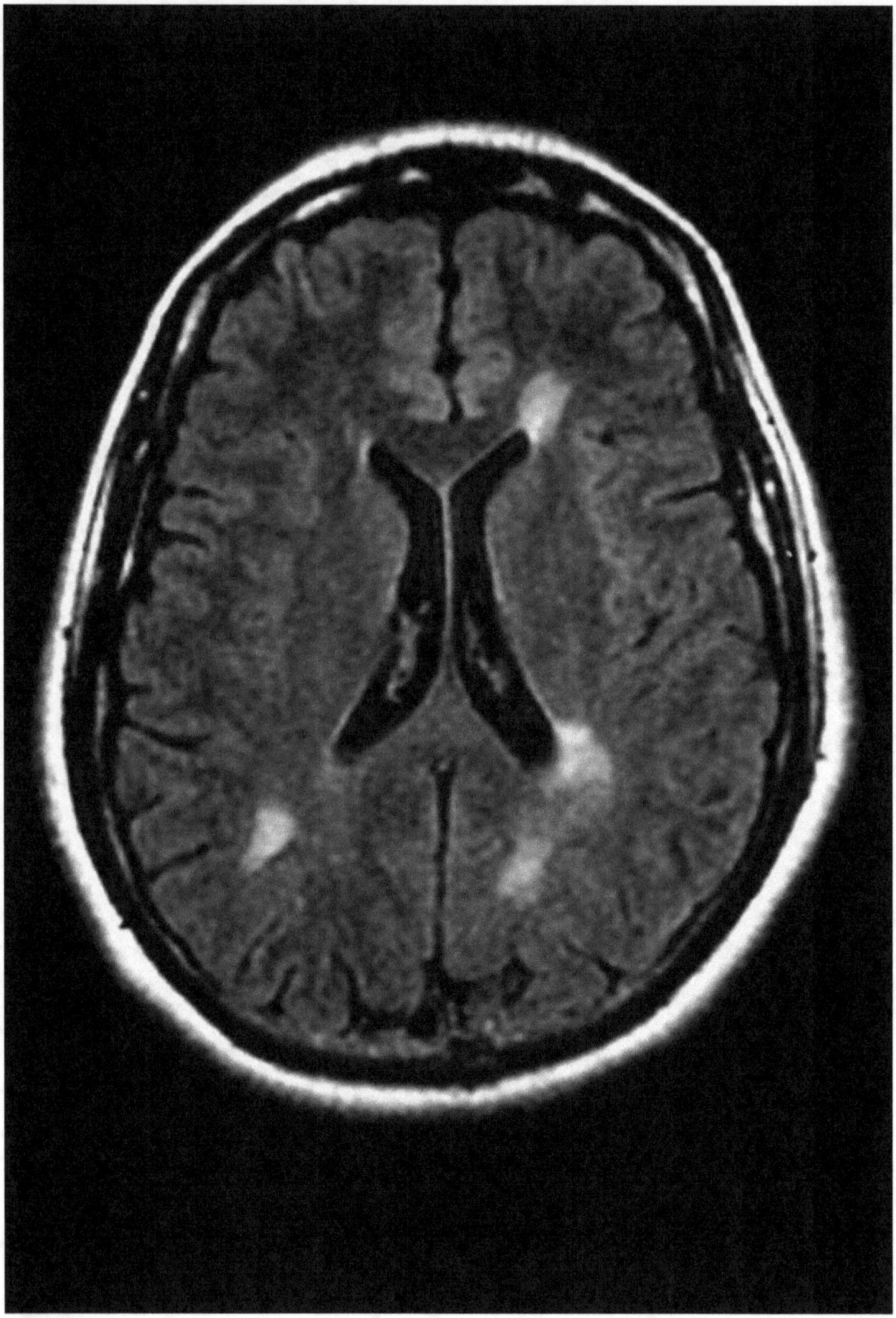

Figure A.6b

Ultrasound

Ultrasound is an imaging technique that uses sound waves to form pictures of tissues or organs of the human body. It is also called ultrasonography or sonography. It is considered a noninvasive imaging technology. The sound waves are with a frequency of more than 20,000 Hz, which is the upper threshold of human hearing.

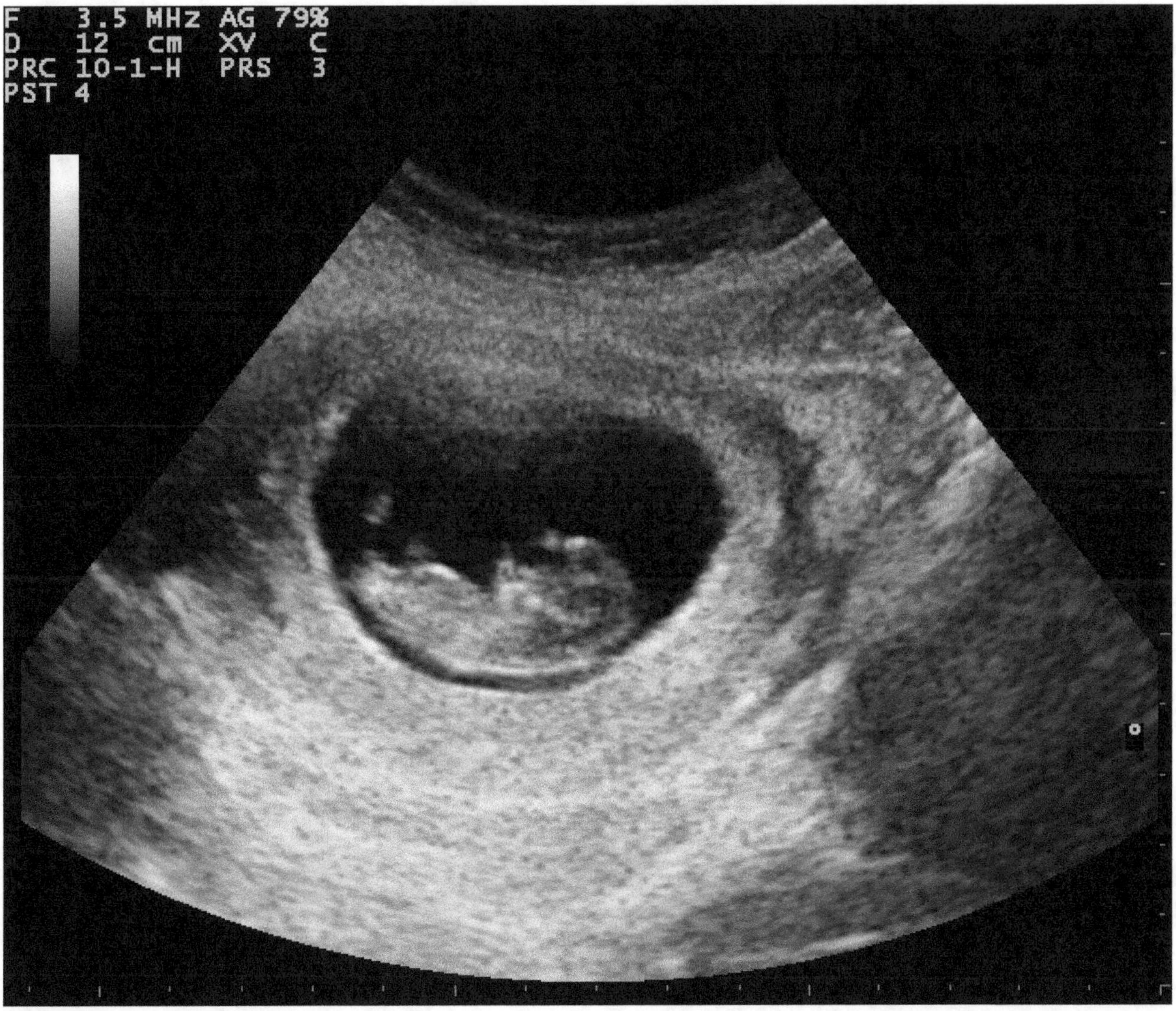

Figure A.7

Endoscopy

Endoscopy is a medical procedure using any type of endoscope, which is a medical device with an attached light and usually the image is transmitted to a screen. An endoscope is composed of an image sensor, optical lens, light source, and mechanical device. The scope is inserted through a natural opening such as bronchoscopy, sigmoidoscopy, anoscopy, and colonoscopy, etc.

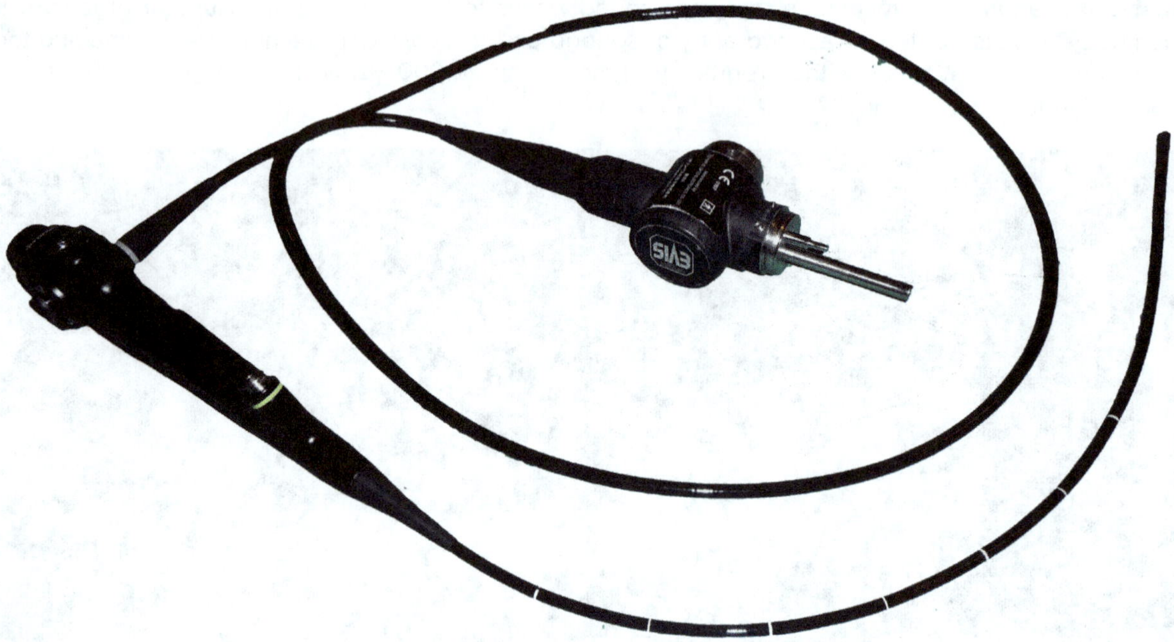

Figure A.8

Cardiac Catheterization

Cardiac Catheterization is a procedure that a catheter is inserted into a large blood vessel in the arm or leg then passes into the heart. The pressure and oxygen levels within the heart can be used to evaluate the heart's function. Through the catheter, a special dye can be injected to create an image of the heart's structure and blood flow condition. When the dye is injected into the three largest coronary arteries, it is called coronary angiography.

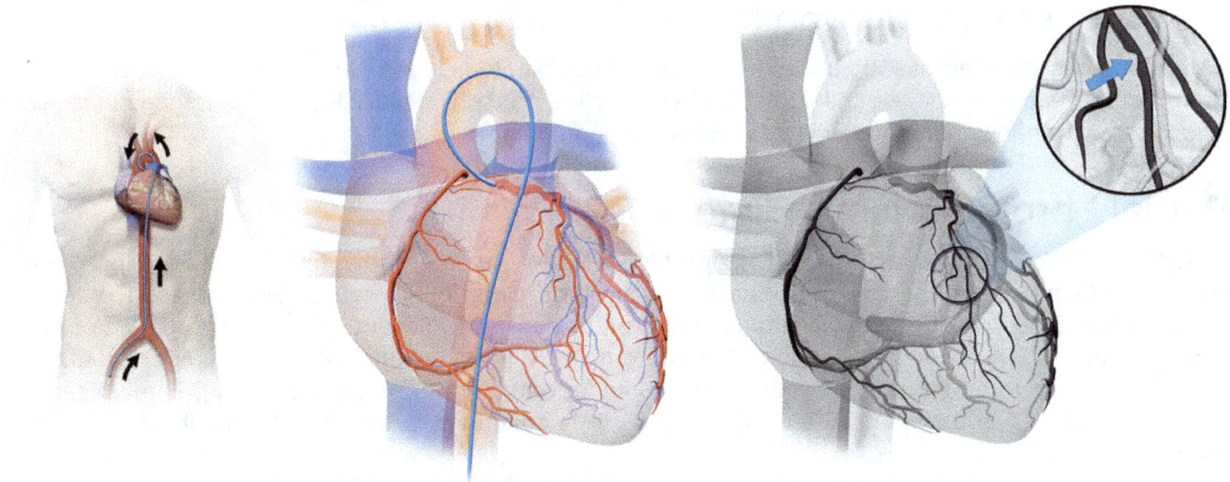

Figure A.9

Complete Blood Count (CBC)

CBC is a blood test. It is used to evaluate the overall health of a person as well as a wide range of conditions including but not limited to anemia, infection, and leukemia. The following things are measured:

- Erythrocyte count: 4.1–5.5 x 10^6/mm^3
- Hematocrit: 37–47%
- Reticulocyte count: 0.5%–1.5%
- Hemoglobin: 12–16 g/dL
- Mean corpuscular volume (MCV): 80–100 fl
- Mean corpuscular hemoglobin (MCH): 27–32 picograms
- Mean corpuscular hemoglobin concentration (MCHC): 30–35 g/dL
- RDW: <15%

CBC with Differential

The CBC differential refers to the subtype white blood cell count.

Leukocyte count: 4,500–11,000/mm^3
Neutrophils: 40%–60%
Lymphocytes: 20%-40%
Monocytes: 4%–8%
Eosinophils: 1%–3%
Basophils: 0%–1%
Bands: 0%–5%

Basic Metabolic Panel (BMP)

BMP is a test that measures eight different substances in the blood. It provides important information about the chemical balance and metabolism in the body. The BMP includes glucose, calcium, sodium, potassium, carbon dioxide, chloride, blood urea nitrogen (BUN), and creatinine.

Comprehensive Metabolic Panel (CMP)

CMP measures 14 different substances from a blood sample. It includes glucose, calcium, sodium, potassium, bicarbonate, chloride, albumin, total protein, alkaline phosphatase (ALP), alanine transaminase (ALT), aspartate aminotransferase (AST), bilirubin, BUN, and creatinine.

Partial Thromboplastin Time (PTT)

PTT, also known as activated PTT (aPTT), is a blood test to measure how long it takes for the blood to clot. The PTT measures the overall speed at which blood clots form through two consecutive series of reactions known as intrinsic pathway and common pathway. The PTT indirectly measures action of the following coagulation factors: I (fibrinogen), II (prothrombin), V (proaccelerin), VIII (anti-hemophilic factor), X (Stuart-Prower factor), XI (plasma thromboplastin antecedent), and XII (Hageman factor). The typical reference range of PTT is between 25 and 33 seconds. It is commonly prescribed to monitor the treatment effect of heparin.

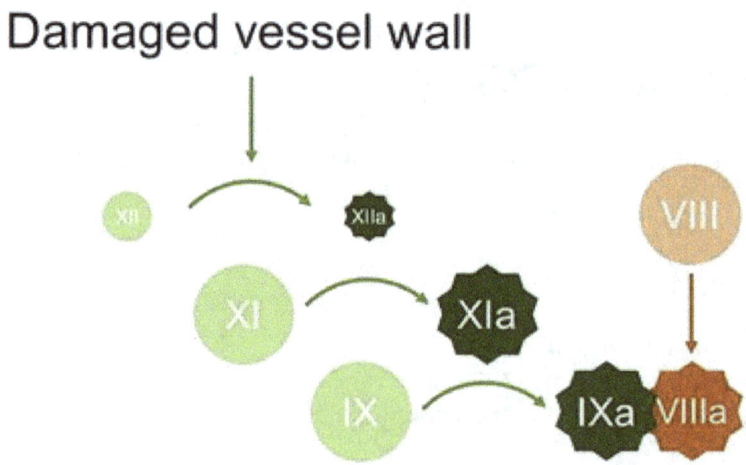

Figure A.10

The **PTT** is often used in conjunction with another measure of how quickly blood clotting takes place, called the prothrombin time (**PT**). The PT measures the speed of clotting by means of the extrinsic pathway and common pathway. An **INR** (international normalized ratio) is a type of calculation based on PT test results. PT measures the following coagulation factors: I (fibrinogen), II (prothrombin), V (proaccelerin), VII (proconvertin), and X (Stuart-Prower factor). The normal range for PT is 12 to 13 seconds. The INR is from 0.8 to 1.2. For patients on anticoagulant treatment, the INR is controlled between 2 and 3.

The **thrombin time (TT)**, also known as the **thrombin clotting time (TCT)**, is measuring the time it takes for a clot to form in the plasma of a blood sample containing anticoagulant, after an excess of thrombin has been added. The normal range is between 12 and 14 seconds. A longer TT can mean a fibrinogen abnormality, impairment of fibrin formation, and/or a thrombin inhibitory effect. It can also be caused by medicine that affect blood clotting, such as heparin or argatroban. It is used to diagnose blood coagulation disorders and to assess the effectiveness of fibrinolytic therapy.

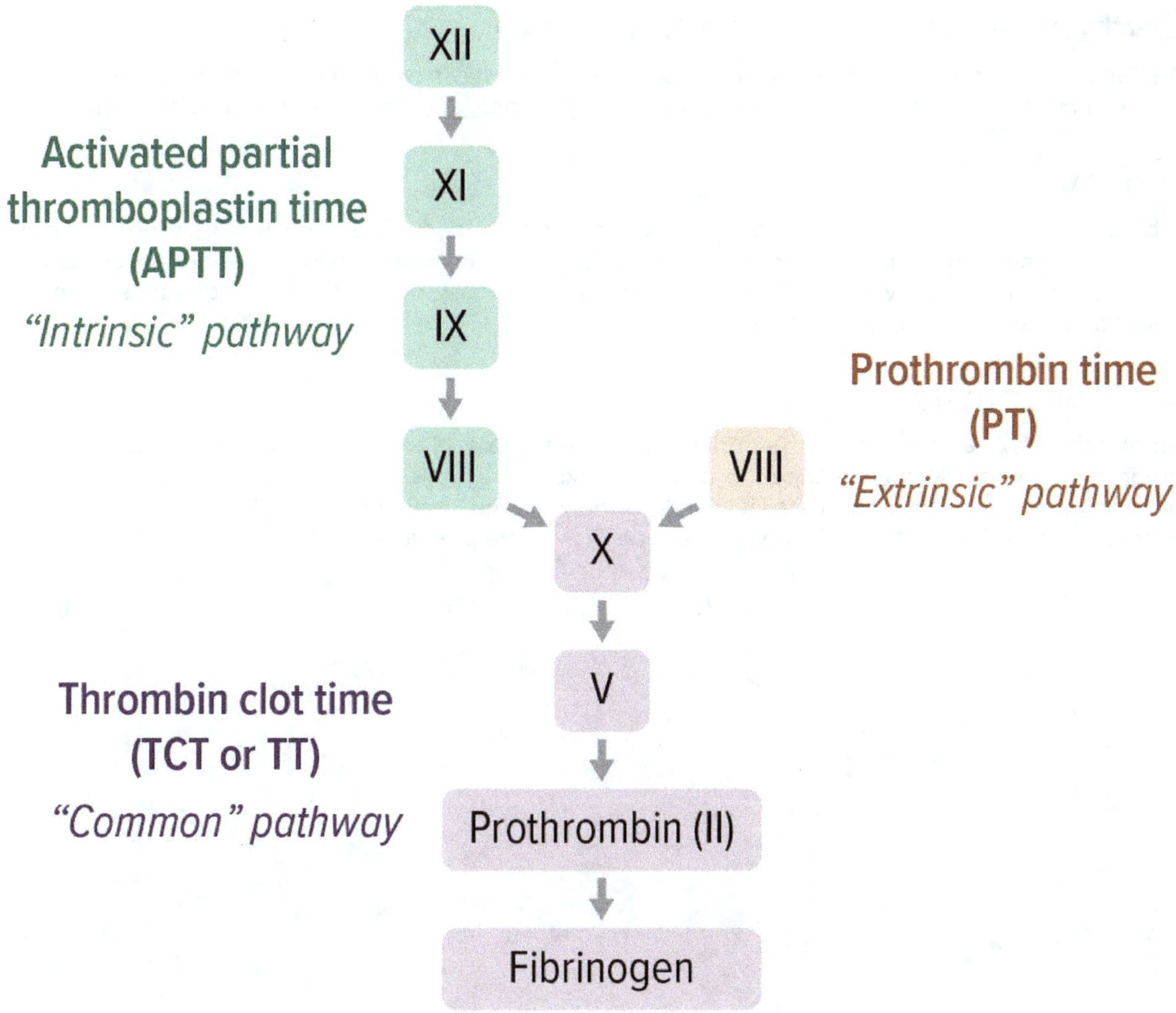

Figure A.11

A1C

A1C is a blood test for measuring the blood glucose level over the previous three months. It is used to diagnose type 2 diabetes or evaluate diabetes management. The test result is given in percentages. The higher the percentage, the higher the blood glucose level.

- A normal A1C is below 5.7%
- 5.7%–6.4%: Prediabetes
- 6.5% or above: Diabetes

D-dimer Test

D-dimer is a protein fragment formed when a blood clot dissolves in the body. The D-dimer test is used to find out whether there is a blood clotting disorder such as deep vein thrombosis (DVT), pulmonary embolism (PE), disseminated intravascular coagulation (DIC), and stroke.

Erythrocyte Sedimentation Rate (ESR)

An **ESR** is a blood test that can show inflammation in the body. It can be used to monitor or diagnose inflammation related conditions including arthritis, vasculitis, infection, and inflammatory bowel disease.

Biopsy

A **biopsy** is a procedure that removes cells or tissues from the body. Then the cells or tissue are used to check for damage or diseases. It includes bone biopsy, bone marrow biopsy, breast biopsy, colposcopy, kidney biopsy, liver biopsy, needle biopsy of the lung, skin biopsy, sentinel lymph node biopsy, chorionic villi sampling, and thyroid needle biopsy.

Amniocentesis

Amniocentesis is a test to diagnose certain genetic disorders, birth defects, or other conditions during pregnancy. It is usually done between 15 and 20 weeks of pregnancy. It is commonly used to 1) diagnose genetic and chromosomal disorders including down syndrome, cystic fibrosis, sickle cell disease, or Tay-Saches disease; 2) detect neural tube defects; and 3) evaluate premature birth risk.

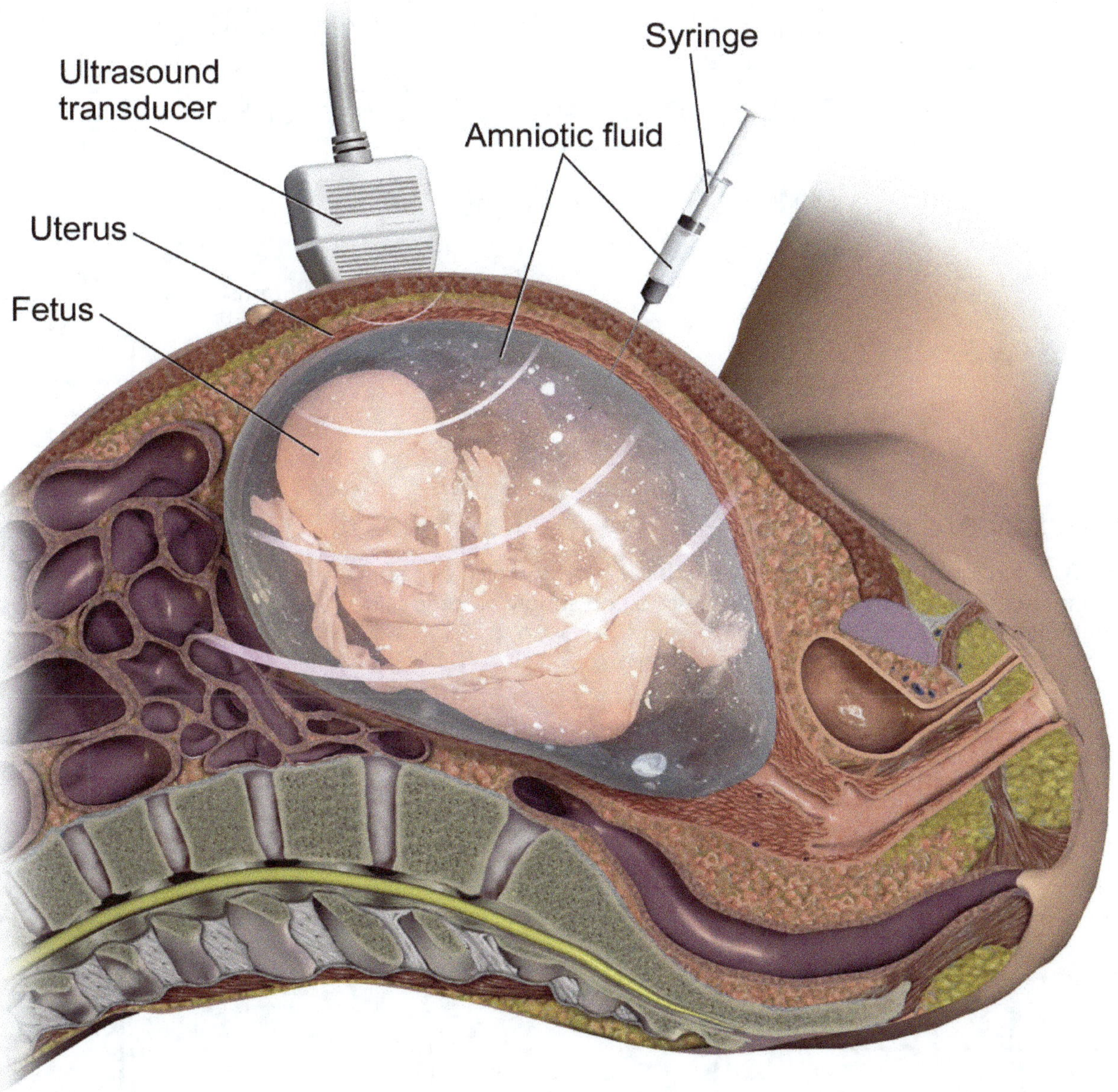

Figure A.12

Electroencephalogram (EEG)

An **EEG** is the electrical activity of the brain is recorded by electrodes placed on the scalp. The signal was collected and shown on a screen. The EEG may be recommended to help diagnose epilepsy, encephalopathy, encephalitis, sleep disorders, or some developmental disorders.

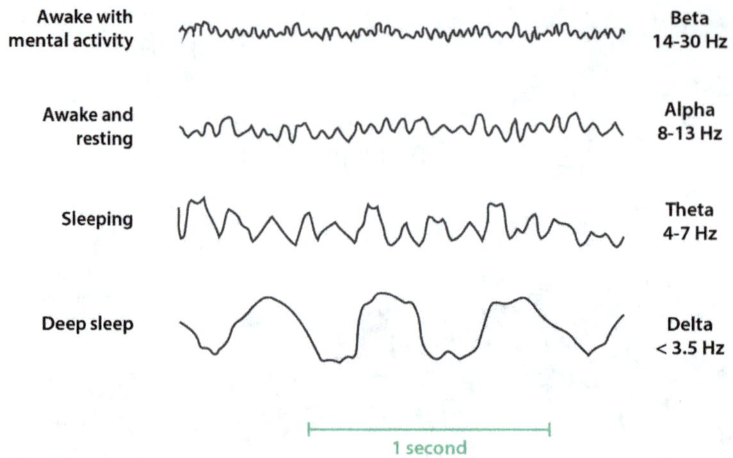

Figure A.13

Electrocardiogram (ECG)

An **ECG** is a recording of the heart's electrical activity, which can show whether a person is having or has had a heart attack, a stressed heart due to blood supply blockade, irregular heart rhythms, pericarditis, or abnormal heart electrical pathways.

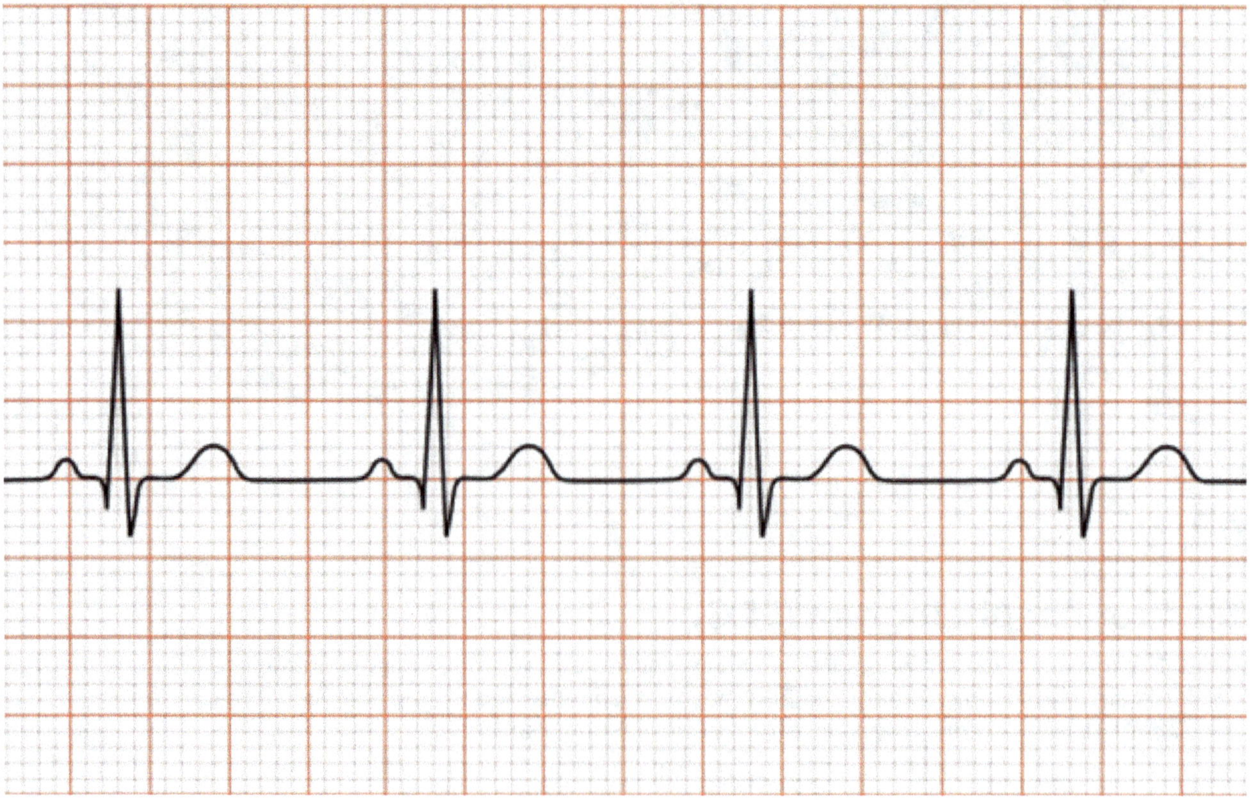

Figure A.14

Image Credits

Fig. A.1: Copyright © 2017 Pixabay/Taokinesis.

Fig. A.2: Copyright © 2017 Pixabay/AlarconAudiovisual.

Fig. A.3: Copyright © 2018 Pixabay/OsloMetX.

Fig. A.4a: Copyright © 2008 by Jon Callas (CC BY 2.0) at https://www.flickr.com/photos/joncallas/2892615027.

Fig. A.4b: Copyright © 2015 by Journal of Diagnostic Imaging in Therapy (CC BY-SA 2.0) at https://www.flickr.com/photos/jdit/16439840070.

Fig. A.5: Copyright © 2021 Depositphotos/Wirestock.

Fig. A.6a: Copyright © 2013 Depositphotos/sudok1.

Fig. A.6b: ISM/SOVEREIGN, "Multiple Sclerosis Lesions," Multiple Sclerosis News Today, https://multiplesclerosisnewstoday.com/ms-lesions/. Copyright © 2022 by Bionews, Inc.

Fig. A.7: Copyright © 2010 by Nevit Dilmen (CC BY-SA 3.0) at https://commons.wikimedia.org/wiki/File:Pregnancy_ultrasound_110322105347_1056300.jpg.

Fig. A.8: Copyright © 2009 by Håkon Olav Leira (CC BY-SA 3.0) at https://commons.wikimedia.org/wiki/File:Bronkoskop.jpg.

Fig. A.9: Copyright © 2017 by BruceBlaus (CC BY-SA 3.0) at https://commons.wikimedia.org/wiki/File:Coronary_Angiography.jpg.

Fig. A.10: Screenshot from Medmastery, https://www.youtube.com/watch?v=wSlkGgBsvkY, 2018.

Fig. A.11: Adapted from Howard M. Reisner, Pathology: A Modern Case Study. Copyright © 2015 by McGraw-Hill Education.

Fig. A.12: Copyright © 2015 by BruceBlaus (CC BY-SA 4.0) at https://commons.wikimedia.org/wiki/File:Amniocentesis.png.

Fig. A.13: Shruthi Sivakumar, https://www.firstclassmed.com/articles/2017/eeg-waves. Copyright © 2017 by Firstclass.

Fig. A.14: British Heart Foundation, https://www.bhf.org.uk/-/media/images/information-support/tests/ecg/normal-ecg-620×400.jpg.

www.ingramcontent.com/pod-product-compliance
Lightning Source LLC
LaVergne TN
LVHW080050210926
848481LV00011B/3317